ANNE CHARLISH is a medi_____ ___ ___ _____ in making complex medical _____ _____ __ the general reader. Her previous books include *First Aid and Home Safety*, *Home Security* and *The Damart Guide for Back Pain Sufferers*. Anne Charlish also writes consumer and fashion features for women's magazines such as *Homes & Gardens* and articles and books on aspects of horses and horsemanship.

DR BRIAN GAZZARD did his medical training at Cambridge and then went to King's College Hospital in London. After doing a variety of junior hospital doctor's jobs he did his gastroenterological training at the Liver Unit at King's College Hospital and at the Gastro enterological Unit of St Bartholomew's Hospital. He became a consultant at St Stephen's and Westminster Hospitals in 1978. He is married with three children.

Overcoming Common Problems Series

Overcoming Common Problems Series

Overcoming Common Problems Series

Overcoming Common Problems

HOW TO CURE YOUR ULCER

Anne Charlish
and Dr Brian Gazzard

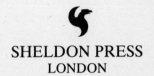

SHELDON PRESS
LONDON

First published in Great Britain in 1988 by
Sheldon Press, SPCK, Marylebone Road, London NW1 4DU

British Library Cataloguing in Publication Data

Charlish, Anne
    How to cure your ulcer.
    1. Man. Gastrointestinal tract. Peptic
    ulcers
    I. Title   II. Gazzard, Brian   III. Series
    616.3′43

    ISBN 0–85969–571–9

Photoset by Deltatype Ltd, Ellesmere Port
Printed in Great Britain by Richard Clay Ltd, Bungay, Suffolk

To Dr John Cutting, whose inspiration this book was.

Contents

Introduction

by Dr Brian Gazzard

One of the most important changes to have taken place in medicine over the last 30 years or so is that many doctors now believe that the more the patient knows about his or her illness, the better. It used to be felt that medicine should be a magic art which was not open to patients to understand and that they should merely obey their doctor's instructions in order to get better. This was in the days when the doctors really had very few effective remedies and the placebo effect of the doctor's personality and reassurance was therefore important in the treatment of many diseases. Now, however, effective remedies for many common ailments and serious diseases are available and so the need for secrecy on the doctor's part has diminished. Furthermore, doctors are often involved in complex and precise judgements in which the benefits of any form of treatment have to be weighed against its potential toxicity and other side-effects. Clearly, the patient's own preference is important in this equation and he or she has a perfect right to know what major problems may be created by a necessary operation or course of tablets. However, a consultant may have trained and practised medicine every day for more than 20 years and terms and concepts which are immediately familiar to him or her are mumbo-jumbo to the patient.

Many doctors find it difficult to put concepts in terms simple enough to be readily understood by the patient. It is also very difficult for the patient to see himself or herself as a statistic and, therefore, while the consultant may talk to him or her about the chances of an operation being successful, what the patient really wants to know is what will happen in his or her own case.

It is well recognized that a consultation is a time of great

1

stress for the patient, who will often leave the doctor's surgery without a clear impression of all the things the doctor said. Many studies have shown that when the patient talks to relatives half an hour later, he or she can remember little about the consultation and will completely deny being told certain things which were in fact made clear at the time. Two points of advice are therefore important. If possible take someone with you to an important consultation: that person will often be able to remember things much more clearly than you because he or she is less stressed.

Second, have a list of questions that you would like answered before leaving the consultation room. Many doctors do not like being presented with a list of symptoms because they prefer to be able to rely on an overall impression of the problem rather than to be presented with a series of facts, all with equal emphasis. I often feel that if a patient cannot remember about a certain symptom till afterwards, it was probably not a very important part of the problem in the first place. However, I am always happy when patients bring a series of queries to the surgery because that means they tend to leave with a better understanding of the matters which are of concern to them.

One of the problems for the patient is that there is a dearth of good books on health problems which are up to date and yet written in a simple and fairly straightforward style. Going to the library and getting a medical dictionary out is virtually useless as the text is often written in an obscure way, and is usually many years out of date. Self-help books such as the present one are invaluable, therefore, as up-to-date guides written by a lay person so that they are easy to understand.

We are in an era of self-help in which many patients are turning from conventional medicine and looking to healthy living as a way out of many of their medical problems. This approach is to be encouraged and there is no doubt that medical science is increasingly appreciating that a positive attitude to many serious illnesses has a pronounced influence on recovery. A patient's adjustment to a serious disability is also much enhanced if he or she can be encouraged to form part of the decision-making process leading to surgery or to a course of toxic medication.

'Holistic medicine' is a term often used to distinguish the self-help approach from conventional medicine as we know it in the Western world. Such terminology is misleading as holistic medicine implies treating the whole person, but any conventional doctor worth his salt would wish to do this whatever system of medicine he is practising. An important part of this approach to the whole person is giving the patient an adequate and detailed explanation of his or her disease and its treatment.

This book describes what an ulcer is and how it is caused. As a result of my interest in the book I have been asking patients recently about their concept of what an ulcer is, and, although I shouldn't have been surprised, I was, by the very bizarre answers I sometimes received. I hope that reading this book will give you a clear picture of what an ulcer is, how it is caused and what investigations you are likely to undergo if you have an ulcer. A clear chapter on treatment gives a comprehensive review of the treatments presently available, and the difficult decisions associated with the decision to operate. Mention is also made of the drugs that may soon become available.

Old wives' tales with regard to ulcers abound. They are commonly thought to be a disease of the professional stressed classes, made much worse by alcohol and eating chillies, amenable to strict changes in diet and a sign of cancer. None of these beliefs is, in reality, borne out of the evidence, as I hope is made crystal clear in the text.

One of the greatest advances in gastroenterology over the last 20 years has undoubtedly been the introduction of effective treatments for ulcers and there is now no reason why anybody should suffer long-term from indigestion as the result of an ulcer. Self-help in this situation largely means rapid referral to the general practitioner, with the right sort of symptoms being investigated, if necessary, and having the right treatment. Self-help is important in assisting the doctor in making the diagnosis, appreciating the need for futher investigations and remembering to take the entire course of drugs exactly as prescribed.

It is obviously not possible to discuss ulcer symptoms without also discussing other complaints unconnected with ulcers but often mistaken for them, and this is the subject of Chapter 1. Pain in and around the stomach may make you jump to conclusions which turn out to be unjustified and it is advisable, if you are in any doubt, always to go and see your doctor. He or she will often be able to make the correct diagnosis by asking a few simple questions. If he or she does decide to investigate you further, these tests are safe and no more than a little unpleasant, particularly if you have read this book and have a fairly clear idea of what is involved.

1

What Does an Ulcer Feel Like?

There are a number of causes of pain in and around the stomach, and ulcers are only one of these, albeit a fairly common one. People quite often jump to the conclusion that their particular sort of stomach pain is due to an ulcer, however. In this chapter, Dr Brian Gazzard, consultant physician at St Stephen's Hospital, London, discusses the cases of seven people who have consulted him in his outpatients clinic. Their case histories provide us with valuable insights into the kinds of symptom that people with ulcers may experience and some of the conditions that may be confused with ulcers.

Peptic ulcers

Mrs Emily Shepherd is aged 50 and works part time as a hospital cleaner. The following is an extract from her consultation.

Mrs Shepherd: I've had no serious illnesses before but, every so often, for the last five years or so, I've been getting tummy ache. Every time I was about to go and see the doctor about it, the pain got better and I thought I'd wait and see what happened.

Doctor: Whereabouts is the pain?

Mrs Shepherd: (*pointing with one finger*) Right here, at the top of the tummy, just above my waistband. Occasionally the pain goes through to the back but not very often.

Doctor: Does the pain wake you at night?

Mrs Shepherd: Yes, over the last few weeks, I've been waking up at about 4 o'clock every morning with bad stomach ache. I get up and make myself a cup

	of tea and eat some biscuits and the pain seems to go away.
Doctor:	Is the pain usually related to eating or not?
Mrs Shepherd:	Yes, the pain seems to come on when I'm hungry so, providing I eat regularly and have snacks in between, it's not so bad.
Doctor:	Have you been vomiting at all?
Mrs Shepherd:	I'm not usually sick but sometimes I feel as if I'm going to be. One night last week I did bring up quite a lot of horrible tasting stuff but after this the pain went away for a while.
Doctor:	Is the pain usually worse in the morning or the evening?
Mrs Shepherd:	I'm not usually too bad first thing in the morning, but the pain seems to get worse during the day.
Doctor:	Have you lost any weight?
Mrs Shepherd:	No, it's about the same. In fact, I find it very difficult to lose weight at the moment because I feel more comfortable if I'm eating plenty.
Doctor:	Do you smoke?
Mrs Shepherd:	Yes . . . I'm afraid I smoke about fifty cigarettes a day.

Mrs Shepherd gives a very typical history of a *peptic* ulcer. The pain is always in the upper region of the tummy in what is known as the *epigastrium*. If the pain is felt elsewhere in the stomach, the pain is unlikely to be due to ulceration. This pain sometimes goes through to the back and this may be a sign that the ulcer is quite deep, and irritating the organ that lies behind the stomach which is called the *pancreas*.

Although such pain typically comes on immediately after a meal, or when the patient is hungry, about half of those who have a peptic ulcer and consult a specialist don't notice any relationship between eating food and the development of the pain. However, it is characteristic for the pain to be intermittent, lasting for an hour or two at a time, rather than be present throughout the day. Ulcers tend to heal and break down in a cyclical fashion, and the fact that the patient gets better for a while often delays their going to the doctor.

It is believed that the pain of an ulcer is caused by acid in the stomach. Food tends to buffer this acid, so the pain may often get better for a few hours after eating a meal. However, by the middle of the night there is no food left in the stomach and so the patient wakes with pain. By the morning, the stomach hasn't been stimulated with any food for many hours and therefore the acid production is at its lowest. Therefore, interestingly, first thing in the morning, the patient is often quite well and has no pain.

Mrs Shepherd is typical of ulcer sufferers in that she smokes. There is no doubt that smokers are more likely to get ulcers than non-smokers and it is more difficult to heal such ulcers.

Finally, it's an old wives' tale that ulcers are common in the professional classes. Even if manual workers like Mrs Shepherd do not smoke, they're much more likely to get ulcers than other groups of society.

Complications

Perforated ulcers

Mr Miller is in his late fifties and is head of the history department at his local school. He has been taking painkillers for several years, while awaiting a hip-replacement operation. Dr Gazzard asks Mr Miller to tell him about this first.

Mr Miller: For the last four years I've had a lot of trouble with my right hip. Unfortunately, there's a long waiting list for replacements and so I've had to make do with painkillers. I've tried a whole variety of drugs which my doctor tells me are called non-steroidal anti-inflammatory drugs. Very occasionally I've had a bit of indigestion which has settled very quickly when I've taken a Rennies tablet.

However, on the whole, I've been very well until last night when at 3 o'clock in the morning I woke up with a terrible pain which went through to my back and made me sweat. The pain started in the upper part of the stomach and quite rapidly spread over the whole of the stomach area. I'm still in considerable pain now, although I've had an injection to help me.

Doctor: Are you still taking tablets for your hip?

Mr Miller: Yes, the pain has been very bad in my hip and I've been taking eight tablets a day.

Doctor: Have you had your bowels open today?

Mr Miller: No, I haven't.

Doctor: Have you been able to pass any wind?

Mr Miller: Well, I haven't passed any wind down below for the last twenty-four hours.

Doctor: Are you able to stand up?

Mr Miller: No, every time I try to stand I feel very faint and have to lie down again.

Doctor: I'm sorry to say that it looks as though the tablets you've taken have produced an ulcer either in the stomach or in the duodenum, which is the bit of the intestine connected to the stomach. I think this ulcer has probably eroded right through the wall of your stomach and is producing peritonitis. I think you'll have to have an operation in the next few hours, but don't worry because I'm sure you'll soon be well – this operation is quite simple and straightforward.

Mr Miller's is a classic case of a peptic ulcer which is

perforated. This produces peritonitis and nearly always requires an operation. Very occasionally, if you're at sea or in other circumstances where no experienced surgeon is available, you might be treated by putting a tube down into your stomach to suck out all the gastric juice; you would also be unable to eat, and would be fed instead via a vein. However, an operation is nearly always performed to sew up the hole in the stomach and to cleanse the abdominal cavity. Sometimes, an operation is performed at the same time to prevent the ulcer recurring, but at other times, if the patient is very ill, the ulcer is just sewn up. Definitive treatment is left until later.

A variety of drugs, which are all called non-steroidal, anti-inflammatory drugs, and which are now used to treat arthritic pains, all seem to cause ulceration. These drugs relieve the pain of arthritis by inhibiting the production of substances called *prostaglandins* which are important in producing an inflammatory response. These prostaglandins are probably also important in protecting the stomach from attack by acid and so, if a patient is taking the drugs, the stomach may become damaged and an ulceration caused.

As in Mr Miller's case, it is often common to have very little trouble from an ulcer before it actually perforates. The incidence of perforation, particularly in elderly ladies taking these drugs, is quite high and is causing a lot of concern, particularly as many patients take these drugs when they in fact have very little pain.

Perforation used to be a very common complication of peptic ulceration, but in recent years the incidence of perforation has fallen very considerably. It is not clear whether this is because fewer people are developing peptic ulcers or whether modern treatments have made perforation of an ulcer less likely.

Bleeding

Peter Metcalfe is a 23-year-old assembly worker in a car factory.

Mr Metcalfe:	I've had indigestion off and on for about four years. Yesterday morning, though, I suddenly felt quite faint and I had slight diarrhoea and then half an hour later vomited half a basin full of blood.
Doctor:	Can you describe the motion a little more exactly?
Mr Metcalf:	It was sticky and black a bit like tar and blood seemed to ooze out of it.
Doctor:	Had you been taking any aspirins or other tablets?
Mr Metcalfe:	No.
Doctor:	Did you know what the cause of the indigestion was?
Mr Metcalfe:	Well, about three years ago I went to have a barium meal which showed a duodenal ulcer. I'd taken some tablets from my GP which cured the problem. When this was happening I had been having some further stomach pains. I decided to go back to the GP and get some more tablets.
Doctor:	Obviously, you do have a peptic ulcer and this has damaged one of the arteries in the stomach which is leaking blood, causing it to appear both in the stool and in the stomach from which it was vomited. We obviously need to replace some of the blood and try and give you some medicine to heal the ulcer as quickly as possible. Most people stop bleeding quite quickly but occasionally the bleeding goes on. You would then require an operation to tie off the artery.

Ulcer bleeding is quite an uncommon but nevertheless very frightening complication of having a peptic ulcer. Bleeding may occur because small blood vessels (*capillaries*) are damaged and blood oozes into the stomach. The bleeding nearly always stops fairly quickly. Alternatively, it can occasionally occur because a big artery is eroded, in which case the bleeding may be massive. Bleeding is perhaps more likely to occur if an irritant compound such as aspirin is taken.

Although bleeding is very frightening, the patient usually recovers very quickly. Obviously, younger patients are more resilient than older ones. In the case of old people who have had a very massive haemorrhage, probably the safest thing to do is to have an operation as soon as possible to make sure that no more bleeding occurs. In the case of younger patients it is better to wait, if possible, as the ulcer can usually be persuaded to heal by medical means.

Pyloric stenosis

Mr Edward Sands is aged 70. He has already had a duodenal ulcer and suffers indigestion.

Mr Sands:	I've had indigestion for as long as I can remember . . . it comes and goes and I often have symptoms for a month or more and then it disappears for three or four months.
	I did have a barium meal about five years ago which showed that I had an ulcer in the duodenum and when I have the indigestion the doctor gives me some tablets called cimetidine which cure it. Anyway, about three weeks ago I started to vomit. I would eat a meal and quite suddenly, with no apparent effort, I would be sick. Quite often I'd notice things in the vomit which I had eaten two or three days before like tomato skins.
Doctor:	Does the vomit dribble out of your mouth or does it come out forcibly?
Mr Sands:	Well, it seems to pump out everywhere, and

11

	sometimes it goes in a stream of quite a distance.
Doctor:	Do you have any indigestion at present?
Mr Sands:	No, funnily enough, I have been fairly free of indigestion for the last few months and so I was quite surprised when I started being sick.
Doctor:	You have a condition called pyloric stenosis. This is a condition in which the outlet to the stomach becomes narrow as a result of the healing process from the ulcer that you have had in your duodenum. We are unable to treat this with drugs and we need to make a separate drainage hole in your stomach. This is a simple operation and you should feel a lot better afterwards.

Pyloric stenosis is quite a rare complication of peptic ulceration, but we have no way of treating it medically and a simple operation is always required to relieve the obstruction. We do not know whether or not keeping the patient completely symptom-free by continuing to prescribe him or her with drugs which heal the ulcer will prevent this complication from occurring.

Other causes of stomach pain

Irritable bowel syndrome

Miss Diane Roberts is a secretary aged 23. She has been suffering stomach ache, often combined with a sense of bloatedness, for several years.

Miss Roberts:	For as long as I can remember I have had tummy ache. Sometimes, I get pain low down in the tummy which is griping and may last for two or three days. But I also get pain in the top

part of the tummy which very occasionally wakes me at night and I sometimes think it's related to food but not always. My stomach gets bloated quite often and it sometimes looks as though I am nine months pregnant. I get lots of wind at both ends.

Doctor: What about your bowel action?

Miss Roberts: I have lots of diarrhoea, particularly when the pain is bad.

Doctor: What do you mean by diarrhoea?

Miss Roberts: Well, in the morning, I can't get out of the house for an hour or two because I keep wanting to go to the lavatory, with acute diarrhoea. Every time I go to the lavatory I don't feel completely empty and have to go again.

Doctor: Is the stool completely liquid or is it formed within lots of bits and pieces?

Miss Roberts: It's often in lots of little bits and pieces rather like rabbit droppings.

Doctor: When you go to the lavatory, does the griping pain get better?

Miss Roberts: Yes, for a short while, but then it comes back.

Doctor: If you pass wind does the bloating and tummy pain get better?

Miss Roberts: Yes.

Doctor: Do you have any particular worries in your life at the moment?

Miss Roberts: I have always been a highly strung person but I have had a lot of trouble recently because my boyfriend wants to marry me but I'm not sure that's the right thing to do.

Doctor: Do you think that stress may have anything to do with your pain?

Miss Roberts: I sometimes think that it might.

This is a common history which may be very difficult to sort out. The most important symptom here may be due to a condition called 'irritable bowel syndrome' in which spasms in the bowel cause pain and often lead to diarrhoea with unusual stool forms. Relief of the pain by going to the lavatory is a sure sign that the pain comes from the colon rather than the stomach. Such patients often do have a lot of stress.

This condition is very common and may affect 10 to 15 per cent of the population. Peptic ulcer is also very common and between 5 and 10 per cent of people can expect to have an ulcer at some time in their life – it is quite common to get both conditions together.

Because of this, the doctor sometimes finds it very difficult to be certain whether or not there is some disease other than irritable bowel syndrome causing the symptoms. Obviously, stressed people can get ulcers, although it's an old wives' tale that stress itself tends to produce ulcers. I think in this sort of situation the doctor will tend to investigate the patient, both to reassure him or her that there was no major problem and also to make sure that no ulcer was present.

Irritable bowel syndrome is so common – some one in ten people suffer daily with it – that it's worth mentioning here how to alleviate it. It may respond to increasing the amount of fibre in the stool, either by a change in diet (by eating more whole grains in the form of granary bread and brown pasta, and more vegetables) or by taking a proprietary bulking agent (for example Isogel or Regulan). Sufferers can, in addition, take an anti-spasmodic such as mebeverene (sold as Colofac) to relieve pain. There is little doubt that the pain is often worse at periods of great anxiety and I believe that relaxation exercises and other methods to reduce stress help with this condition.

Gallstones

Mrs Dorothy Harris is a 51-year-old mother of five.

Mrs Harris: About two years ago I started to get quite

severe pain in the upper part of the tummy which lasted about two or three days at a time. I have had to call the doctor out on a couple of occasions because the pain has been so bad. I think that I've sometimes had a temperature with the pain and I've also put on quite a bit of weight in recent years.

Doctor:	Does the pain go anywhere else or is it always in the centre of the tummy?
Mrs Harris:	Sometimes it seems to go over to the right side a bit and quite often I feel a pain in the middle of the back with it.
Doctor:	Have you noticed any change in the colour of the stools or the urine when you get the pain?
Mrs Harris:	Yes, on one occasion my urine appeared a very dark yellow brown and my stools were putty coloured for a couple of days.
Doctor:	At that time did you notice that you were jaundiced?
Mrs Harris:	No.

This is not the story of a peptic ulcer. The pain is not typical of an ulcer – it sounds more like gallstones. Because the blood's waste products are not excreted through the obstructed bile ducts, they are excreted instead in the urine which becomes very dark. The patient may or may not associate this with jaundice. Sometimes the patient may have a temperature and quite frequently he or she goes to Casualty or has to call the doctor out because the pain is so severe. Gallstones are said to be commoner in fat, fertile women of fifty but it is a possible diagnosis at any age.

Heartburn

Mrs Doreen Williamson is a 53-year-old clerk with the local council. Like Mrs Harris, Mrs Williamson has also been overweight for some years, a problem aggravated by the sedentary nature of her job.

15

Mrs Williamson:	I get a burning pain in the lower part of my chest and upper part of my tummy when I eat a heavy meal.
Doctor:	Are there any other conditions which bring this on?
Mrs Williamson:	What do you mean?
Doctor:	Does bending over to do your shoes up or pick something up from the floor bring on the pain?
Mrs Williamson:	Yes, I have noticed that when I bend over I get a burning pain in the lower part of my chest and I sometimes also feel a sensation of acid in the back of my throat.
Doctor:	Do you also get the pain when you lie down at night?
Mrs Williamson:	Yes, particularly when I lie on my right side and also if I go to bed soon after a heavy meal.
Doctor:	Do you find any difficulty actually swallowing the food?
Mrs Williamson:	No, not really, but I sometimes feel very full after quite a small meal.

Again, this is not a story of a peptic ulcer but one of heartburn. Heartburn is a rather ill-defined term used by patients to mean a burning pain low in the chest or in the upper part of the tummy which may be associated with eating. There is often a lot of wind which passes upwards (*eructation*) which may relieve the symptoms. Sometimes, no obvious sign of disease in any particular part of the body is found in such patients but more usually they have a hiatus hernia. This means that the muscle separating the stomach from the chest cavity has become rather loose and allowed the little knuckle of stomach to slip upwards into the chest. This allows acid normally contained in the stomach to slide up and down the gullet, causing an inflammation. The patient may notice this as acid comes into the back of the throat. The treatment may be quite similar to that for a peptic ulcer, but the patient often responds less well.

Dr Gazzard's seven patients give an idea of the different conditions that could be confused, by the patient, with an ulcer and its complications, and the difficulties of diagnosis. The next chapter defines and describes an ulcer, and the possible complications.

2
What Ulcers Are

An ulcer is a break in any body surface, internal or external, that heals only with difficulty. There are different types, occurring in the mouth, the eye, on the legs or elsewhere on the body, but the kind I want to deal with are called *peptic* ulcers, which most of us think of as stomach ulcers. They are named after a substance called pepsin, which, as we shall see later, is crucial to the whole story.

In fact, there are two types of peptic ulcers – those which happen in the stomach, known as gastric ulcers, and those which occur in the duodenum, known as duodenal ulcers. The duodenum is immediately behind the stomach, and forms the first part of the small intestine (see diagram). Duodenal and gastric ulcers have some things in common but not all.

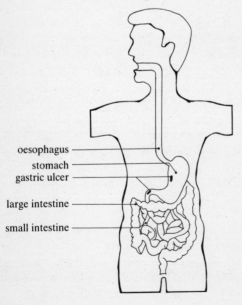

oesophagus

stomach

gastric ulcer

large intestine

small intestine

Ulcers can also occasionally occur in another part of the gut, such as the lower part of the gullet (the oesophagus) which leads down into the stomach. This happens when the valve between the oesophagus and the stomach is not working properly: once food has passed down the oesophagus, the valve should close. If it doesn't, some of the acidic gastric juices may come up the oesophagus and cause heartburn. Although heartburn can herald the presence of oesophagal ulcers, it is more commonly due to inflammation which is not yet so severe that it has progressed to ulceration.

The surface of the gut, or gastrointestinal tract, is nothing like an exterior body surface covered in skin: if you pull down your lower lip and expose the red, slightly sticky material inside your mouth, you will see exactly what the inside of your gut looks like. This material is known as a mucous membrane, a membrane covered with a slightly sticky layer of mucus. An ulcer in the mucous membrane is simply a break or gap in the surface. Some of these breaks heal of their own accord, but they often fail to do so because the acid contained in the gastric juices, which is essential to break down food, keeps working on the breach and so preventing it from healing.

The body can only make use of the food it takes in if it is properly broken down. It is then stored for energy and the waste products are expelled in the form of urine and faeces. This breaking down is a continuous process that starts in the mouth and continues down through the body. The digestive juices are stimulated to some extent merely by the sight of food, and the process gathers momentum as the food travels down the oesophagus. When food reaches the stomach, an enzyme known as *pepsin* (after which peptic ulcers are named) is produced. At the same time, the stomach produces a powerful acid. The mixture of pepsin and the gastric acids, is so fierce that if some were spilled on your skin, it would burn it. If you were to leave a razor blade in the mixture overnight, it would dissolve. More practically, the mixture of pepsin and gastric acids is powerful enough to break down almost anything you present it with: raw carrots, tripe and nuts, for example.

Given that the pepsin and acid, together called the gastric juices, are sufficiently strong to reduce almost anything to liquid and loose waste matter, it is surprising that breaks or ulcers in the lining of the gut don't occur more often or that the stomach lining is not itself broken down and digested.

Several things stop this happening. What we've seen so far are the *aggressive* factors in the formation of ulcers, but there are also *defensive* factors to take into account. The first factor is the *mucosal layer*, which lines the gut, whose chemicals protect it from the corrosive effects of the acid. The second is that in a normal person the amount of pepsin, and therefore the acid produced, is about right to digest the food in the stomach. Sometimes, however, the secretion of pepsin, and therefore acid, is far too much and this is one of the causes of ulcers.

There is an inbuilt defence mechanism in the body to prevent ulcers forming: the cells in the stomach which produce the acid are themselves protected by a substance which makes them immune from the effects of their own secretions. To give a rather morbid illustration of this, when someone dies, it is this substance which stops working first and so, because the acids within the body continue working, the body in effect dissolves itself.

So, the fundamental problem that gives the clue to how ulcers are formed is a change in the ratio between the amount of acid formed in the gut and the effectiveness of the mucosal barrier. There may be too much acid produced within a normal gut, or the amount of acid formed may be about right but the gut lining is weak or ineffective.

One of the differences between gastric ulcers and duodenal ulcers is that, although the duodenum has a protective mechanism against too much acid, it is less resilient than that of the stomach. So, when it receives from the stomach food containing far too much acid, it cannot cope and the excess acid succeeds in breaching the lining – the acid literally burns holes in it.

There are a number of other factors that influence the formation of ulcers and experts have still to agree upon the precise mechanism involved. It may be, for example, that some of the body's defence mechanisms are not working properly. Some people may simply have a weak lining to the gut or it could be that the covering mucus is not thick enough to withstand the onslaught of the gastric juices. It's also been suggested that the flow of blood in the mucosal layer is not adequate, perhaps too slow or too thin, for example, and that the regeneration of the cells of the lining is too slow to be useful.

As well as all these factors, there are also several contributory factors which can lead to producing an ulcer. These include your sex (more men than women develop ulcers), whether your close relatives have ulcers (they tend to run in families), your age, where you live, your social class, your blood group, whether you drink alcohol, and whether you smoke (smokers are twice as likely to develop ulcers as non-smokers and, if ulcers do develop, smokers take twice as long in the healing process). These are just some of the contributory factors involved and are described more fully in Chapter 4, which builds up a picture of the people most likely to develop ulcers.

Duodenal ulcers

Ulcers in the duodenum are ten to fifteen times more common than those in the stomach and for every three or four men who develop one, only one woman will do so. While gastric ulcers tend to develop in people over 40, duodenal ulcers can occur from the age of 20 onwards. And there are other differences, too.

As we have seen, the fundamental issues in the development of ulcers are, first, the levels of pepsin and acid produced in the gut and, second, their equilibrium with the resistance of the barrier formed by the mucous membrane. When the food enters the duodenum, now mixed with acidic gastric juices from

the stomach, the acid is normally neutralized by the duodenum's alkaline secretions. Even so, the duodenum's mucous
membrane is still considerably damaged by the onslaught of
acid but the cells normally regenerate within about twenty-four
hours. Now, if the stomach happens to secrete acid without
food being present, the duodenum will clearly receive more
acid than it can cope with. Some people with duodenal ulcers do
have a secretory capacity that is regarded as higher than normal
– in other words, their stomach may secrete acid without food
being present or they may simply produce too much acid.
Confusingly, however, many don't. The explanation could be
that the cells of their mucosal barrier are more sensitive to these
secretions or that the cells are less sensitive to those substances
that inhibit the effects of the secretions. It could also be that
such people secrete more pepsin and, in addition, secrete acid
during the night while asleep. This is a highly complex problem
and one which many experts are currently engaged upon
resolving.

Gastric ulcers

People who develop gastric ulcers – ulcers in the stomach – tend
to have normal or lower than normal capacities for acid
secretion. So, it could be assumed perhaps that their stomach
lining is less resistant to the acid that they produce, rather than
that they produce too much acid in the first place. Gastric ulcers
tend to occur in people from about the age of 40 onwards, and it
is reasonable to assume that the stomach lining deteriorates
with age, just as every other part of the body does. Nevertheless, some acid is required for the formation of ulcers. There
is a rare condition in which no acid is produced at all and
sufferers will never develop ulcers.

In the case of women, age has a particular bearing upon the
development of ulcers. More men than women suffer with
ulcers, of whatever type and at whatever age, but it has been
established that women are more likely to develop gastric ulcers

after the menopause. It has been suggested that the chief female sex hormone, oestrogen, which is produced until the periods stop, plays a part in preventing the development of gastric ulcers. Once the menopause starts, oestrogen levels begin to decrease and it is about this time that women may develop a gastric ulcer.

Complications

Three of the case studies we examined in Chapter 1 were concerned with the more serious complications accompanying ulcers: first, excessive bleeding or *haemorrhage* (Mr Metcalfe was suffering from this condition); second, perforation of the area of the gut lining in which the ulcer is located (Mr Miller was an example of this); and third, a condition known as *pyloric sterosis* in which the pylorus, the stomach outlet leading to the duodenum, becomes obstructed (Mr Sands was suffering from this disorder).

Haemorrhage

You will always find that a slight bleeding takes place from the raw surface of the ulcer but if the ulcer is particularly deep – although it may not have perforated – it may erode into one of the arteries in the wall of the stomach or duodenum. Once this happens, a massive haemorrhage follows. An unmistakable sign of this happening would be if you were to vomit blood, and another sign would be the later appearance of blood in the faeces giving them a black, tarry appearance, both symptoms which Mr Metcalfe experienced. (Signs and symptoms of internal haemorrhage and the appropriate treatment are described fully in Chapters 3 and 5 respectively.)

Perforated ulcer

The lining of the stomach and the duodenum is made up of several layers. An ulcer can deepen if it is not treated so that the erosion or break in the gut lining penetrates one layer after another until, eventually, it perforates the wall of the gut and either breaks into another organ or, if it does not, the gastric juices flow freely, leading to peritonitis. Of all the complications of ulcers, apart from the Zollinger-Ellison syndrome (see next page), this is the most serious. It is so rare in women that it is practically safe to say it's nearly always confined to men. When it happens, as Mr Miller found, the patient is almost unable to move, is very pale, sweats a lot and has a fast pulse combined with a low blood pressure. What happens is that the highly acidic contents of the stomach or the duodenum find their way into the peritoneal cavity. This cavity is essentially the abdominal cavity and the membrane that lines it is called the *peritoneum* – hence peritoneal cavity. In men the peritoneum is a closed sac with no outlet for the expulsion of waste products and so, once undesirable substances have found their way into it – such as highly acidic gastric matter – there is no escape and the cavity reacts accordingly to the hostile matter. The reaction usually takes the form of severe pain all over the abdominal area and the muscles of the abdomen become rigid – and this is why the patient is almost unable to move.

Pyloric stenosis

If you have a cut or wound on an exterior body surface, it eventually heals by means of the body's blood-clotting abilities and by natural regeneration, leaving scar tissue. Ulcers, however, are constantly hampered in their attempts to heal by the continual erosion caused by the acidic gastric juices. However, some scar tissue will sometimes be formed at the base of the ulcer. If the ulcer has formed at the outlet of the stomach (the *pylorus*), through which softened and partly digested food must pass in order to reach first the duodenum and then the remainder of the small intestine, any scar tissue that has formed may block the outlet. This causes the stomach to become very distended and in turn leads to vomiting in an alarming and spectacular fashion: quite a lot of matter may be thrown up and it may issue forth in an arc with considerable force behind it, in much the same way as described by Mr Sands in Chapter 1. The only way to deal with this is to relieve the obstruction with an operation, called a *gastroenterostomy*, in which the stomach is provided with an alternative drainage outlet.

The cancer connection

There are several components to consider in the ulcer-cancer connection. The rare Zollinger-Ellison syndrome is a form of cancer itself, cancer of the pancreas (which is not always malignant), and this causes extensive ulceration.

Most authorities now believe that neither gastric nor duodenal ulcers turn into cancer. However, a gastric cancer may start with similar symptoms to those of an ulcer, and it is only later that its serious nature is discovered – this is discussed more fully at the end of Chapter 5. Gastric, or stomach, cancers are common, while cancer of the duodenum is very rare indeed.

Drug-induced ulcers

Certain drugs, notably aspirin and drugs for the relief of arthritis, can unfortunately cause ulceration of the gut. This was the root of the problem in Mr Miller's case. Trials and testing for new drugs, before they are allowed on to the market, are now so stringent that at least one doctor has remarked: 'If a drug company tried to market aspirin these days, it would never succeed.' Aspirin is an extraordinarily useful drug – but one of its side-effects may be to cause the stomach to bleed and ulcers to develop. This is not a drug, therefore, that can be taken regularly day after day for the relief of pain, except under close medical supervision. The same goes for the non-steroidal anti-inflammatory drugs prescribed for the relief of pain in arthritis.

Preventing ulcers

The more serious and rare complications of duodenal and

gastric ulcers can usually be avoided provided that the ulcer is diagnosed and treated in its early stages. With new and effective drugs on the market, operations are performed less and less often. The warning signs and symptoms of an ulcer, which are described in the next chapter, should never be ignored and you should be sure to consult a specialist, through your GP, as soon as possible.

3

Diagnosing Ulcers

In attempting to diagnose any illness, your doctor has to look out for signs, whether internal or external, of that illness, and ask you about its symptoms. Some symptoms can signal different complaints – you saw in Chapter 1 that stomach pain doesn't necessarily indicate the presence of ulcers – so the doctor often has to piece together several different bits of information before he can tell you with any confidence what you are suffering from. This applies to ulcers as much as to any other complaint: there are a number of signs and symptoms to look out for which, when taken together, make it probable that an ulcer is present.

Pain

This symptom is common to all ulcer sufferers and is the one that is probably most likely to make you visit your doctor. There are two things which distinguish ulcer pain from pain born of other causes. The first of these is that pain due to other complaints tends to be persistent, whereas ulcer pain comes and goes: it is unusual for an ulcer sufferer to be in pain for more than a few hours at a time, except in those rare cases where the ulcer has perforated (see Chapter 2). You might find yourself experiencing pain every day for several weeks, only to find that it will simply go away for no apparent reason and then come back, again for no apparent reason. Another aspect to this is the tendency for ulcer pain to be seasonal – it has been established that spring and autumn are the worst times of the year for ulcer sufferers.

The second distinguishing factor between ulcer pain and other pains is the location of the pain. Ulcers produce pain in the upper stomach around the solar plexus, which you can feel just above your waist – if it occurs elsewhere you may assume that the cause is probably not an ulcer.

It has been thought for many years that ulcer pain becomes worse immediately after a meal or when hungry. In reality, however, about half of all ulcer patients fail to notice any association between the times meals are taken and the pain. This is not, however, to say that there is no association between pain and actual food intake.

Before you go to your doctor with persistent stomach ache, keep a record of the times of day that the pain is at its worst and when you are relatively pain-free, combined with a note of everything you eat and when you eat it. If there is a relationship with food intake, your doctor should spot it. This association with food intake can point positively to the existence of an ulcer; but that does not mean to say that the absence of any such association means that you do not have an ulcer.

It is especially important that you keep a note of any attack of pain during the night. Ulcer pain is likely to wake you at night, whereas many other sorts of pain would not.

Night waking, as it is known, is directly related to eating. When you eat a meal, two things happen. First, the stomach secretes more acid (see Chapter 2) and, second, the food enters the stomach and buffers the acid. As the food disappears into the duodenum, the stomach continues producing acid for a short time since there is a delay in the mechanism that conveys the information to the stomach that no more acid is needed. Because of this delay, and the continued production of acid, you will, if you have an ulcer, experience pain several hours after eating. Some people find that they can get back to sleep after night waking by taking milk and biscuits – these buffer the acid in the stomach. Ulcer sufferers often find that their most comfortable time of day is the morning, and this is because there has been little or no acid production, because they have not eaten, since the evening meal the night before.

You should try to describe the pain to your doctor as exactly as you can, not only where and when but how it feels.

Distinguish if you can between 'sharp', 'dull, aching', 'throbbing' and 'burning'.

Some of us can put up with more pain than others: our individual pain threshold, the limit of pain that we can tolerate, varies and this makes it difficult for doctors to ascertain exactly how bad a particular patient's pain is. Descriptions of pain vary from person to person, even though the pain they describe may be of the same sort. While doctors agree that the experience of pain probably varies in each individual, it is worth knowing that all ulcer pain is of the type known as *visceral* pain.

There are two sorts of pain, the first of which is the sort you feel when you prick your finger. This is known as *somatic* pain. You know where it is, and you are not frightened by it as you know what the cause is. Somatic pain disappears with aspirin or other over-the-counter analgesics.

The second sort of pain is visceral pain (from 'viscera' meaning the intestines or guts). This sort of pain is more difficult to locate precisely; you will feel that it is vaguely in the stomach. You are more likely to be frightened of it and it will not respond to drugs like aspirin (though it is worth noting here that ulcer pain will respond to antacids like Rennies or Milk of Magnesia). It tends to have a somewhat bizarre, emotional quality, and this may be because it is caused by the nerve fibres that control our emotions (the parasympathetic and sympathetic nervous systems), whereas it is the ordinary nerves of the body that deal with somatic pain.

Nausea and vomiting

Ulcer patients often suffer with nausea or vomiting, or both. If this is the only symptom, however, the cause is unlikely to be an ulcer. But if you have nausea and vomiting, together with stomach pain, and when you vomit the pain gets better almost immediately, you can be reasonably sure that you have an ulcer. A simple explanation for this might be that you are bringing up the excess acid from the stomach, thus relieving the breach in the mucosal layer of further irritation (see Chapter 2).

Incessant vomiting is a sign of one of the complications of ulcers, pyloric stenosis, and this has been described by one of the patients interviewed in Chapter 1, Mr Sands. You should seek emergency medical treatment for this condition, for which a simple operation is the only solution.

It is worth noting here that it has been disproved that vomiting indicates that one sort of ulcer is more likely than another. Large studies have shown that it is not possible to tell without fuller investigation.

Loss of appetite

This is an unreliable symptom in diagnosing ulcers: some people avoid eating because of the association with pain, while others eat all the time to reduce the sensation of the pain – the food buffers the acid in the stomach.

Bleeding

Bleeding is a rare complication of ulcers and must be treated as an emergency. Some people notice blood in the vomit, while others have *melaena*, faeces combined with sticky black stuff with blood oozing from it. In either case, the sufferer should be taken to the casualty department of the local hospital without delay. The patient may feel faint if he or she has lost a considerable amount of blood. If you refer back to Chapter 1, you will see that Mr Metcalfe was such a patient.

Seeing your doctor

If you have several of these symptoms, you may well be correct in assuming that you have an ulcer – you should in any event consult your doctor without delay. With conditions such as these, there is nothing to be gained by putting off the visit: the condition is unlikely to go away and it is likely to worsen and perhaps to develop complications. Straightforward ulcers are mostly treated by pills these days, rather than surgery, so treatment will be rather less painful than going to the dentist, for example.

It is not difficult to confuse a number of other conditions with ulcers, so don't be surprised if your doctor pronounces you free of ulcers but suspects any of the following:

gallstones – the pain will be intermittent, severe and come in bouts. The urine may turn a dark yellow. Mrs Harris interviewed in Chapter 1, was such a patient

irritable bowel syndrome – the pain with this condition, described by Miss Roberts in Chapter 1, may be experienced lower down in the stomach than ulcer pain. It will get either better or worse after a visit to the lavatory, neither of which is the case with ulcers.

heartburn – this pain tends to be higher up in the body than ulcer pain. It is usually felt behind the breastbone, halfway down the chest. It commonly occurs after a large meal and after bending down to pick up something from the floor, as Mrs Williamson agreed in Chapter 1. Acid will come up from the stomach into the throat.

angina – this sort of pain tends to have a constricting quality to it. It is more likely to occur in the cold and during exercise or exertion, unlike ulcer pain, and it is unlikely to occur only after eating.

Medical investigations

Your GP may decide to refer you directly to your local hospital's consultant physician or he/she may decide to send you for a barium meal first and, only when that test proves positive, to refer you. Either way, it should be established what condition you are suffering with. You should not accept long-term prescriptions from your GP for ulcers until the proper hospital investigation has been carried out; a short course of treatment which completely resolves your symptoms is safe, however. It is your right to be referred to a hospital consultant for any persistent condition that your GP has failed to resolve or for confirmation/rebuttal of the GP's diagnosis. If you are over

50 and your GP suspects an ulcer, you should be sent for hospital investigation, in order to eliminate the possibility of a gastric cancer.

Barium meal

This sounds disgusting even if you don't know exactly what it is, but happily you only have to take a mouthful of it – not a meal. It is in fact just a mouthful of a thick, white milky substance; it is not pleasant as it is somewhat cloying. It is a little like eating liquid chalk, if you can imagine that. The point of it is that when you are X-rayed, it shows up white in the stomach and helps the doctor to locate any ulcer, which reveals itself as a white niche.

If you are sent for a barium meal, you must neither eat nor drink for 12 hours before your appointment. You should not take any tablets, either. If you are taking essential medication, such as heart pills for angina, insulin, or contraceptive pills, for example, you should consult your doctor for advice.

After you have swallowed the barium meal, you will be asked to take some fizzy tablets in water. These are intended to blow up the stomach, as it would be if you had just eaten; when the stomach is empty, its sides shrink together so that it appears on an X-ray as a slit rather than a large empty vessel.

A doctor who has specialized in radiology will watch on the X-ray the white barium substance making its way through your gullet into the stomach and duodenum. The entire outline of the stomach will become coated in the white substance, thus highlighting any niche or depression in the stomach edge. As ulcers erode into the stomach wall, they can be seen on the X-ray as white niches, in stark contrast to the black of the stomach wall.

One of the limitations of a barium X-ray is that it can be more difficult to see ulcers in the duodenum than it is to see them in the stomach, particularly if the patient has had a duodenal ulcer in the past; yet ulcers are much more common in the duodenum than the stomach. So a barium X-ray is a useful diagnostic test for a stomach ulcer, but the ulcer is less likely to be there.

A further limitation is imposed by any earlier existence of a

32

duodenal ulcer. If you had had a duodenal ulcer some years before, your duodenum would reveal little craters and deformities on an X-ray. The doctor would then find it difficult to discern between these long-distant abnormalities and the signs of new ulcers. Overall, a barium X-ray fails to spot an ulcer at the rate of one in ten; most of these are picked up later by endoscopy.

The alternative to barium

It is possible for a doctor to see into your stomach with the aid of an instrument known as an *endoscope*, and to detect the existence of any ulcers. This diagnostic test is known as an *endoscopy*. If the picture on the barium X-ray is unclear, you may be referred for endoscopy, as this is a more accurate method of diagnosis. If, on the other hand, the barium X-ray shows normal but the typical symptoms of ulcer persist, you may still be referred for endoscopy as a means of making certain that the barium picture was correct.

Why, you may ask, bother with barium at all if endoscopy is more accurate? Some experts do proceed with endoscopy straight away, particularly if the patient is not elderly. Others feel that, since there are very slight risks attached to endoscopic investigation and none to barium X-ray, it is worth starting with the latter. These very slight risks include having to have a light, mild anaesthetic (rather like a pre-med), and the possibility of the endoscope making a hole in the gullet (causing perforation). But how is an endoscopy carried out?

You must neither eat nor drink for about 12 hours before your appointment (although this can be reduced to four hours in an emergency). You will have to exchange your clothes for an operating gown and remove false teeth, contact lenses and all jewellery in the interests of safety. If you are to have an anaesthetic, you will be asked to remove all make-up, including foundation, powder, blusher and lipstick: this is because your condition under anaesthetic must be monitored; if you were to turn blue, signifying something wrong with your breathing, lipstick or blusher could obscure this vital sign.

You may be given a mild anaesthetic, so mild that most patients remain conscious during the endoscopy but can remember nothing about it afterwards. The back of your throat may be sprayed in order to freeze it: this is to facilitate passing the instrument down your throat and gullet into the stomach. If this is done, you must remember not to drink anything at all for about two hours after you come round; you will not be able to swallow properly and there is therefore a risk that any liquid could pass into your lungs.

Increasingly, these days, endoscopic investigations are being carried out with no anaesthetic. The point of the anaesthetic, when it is given, is to make the patient a little sleepy and generally co-operative; it is not because any discomfort is beyond the pain threshold. If you have to return to work the same day, for example, or you have to drive, the investigation can be carried out without anaesthetic. If you are elderly or for any reason likely to be adversely affected by an anaesthetic you may not be offered one.

The endoscope itself is a small telescope-like instrument, usually about the size of a 1p piece in diameter. Smaller ones are available for children and larger ones are available for use with a patient who is bleeding internally (the blood would obscure the picture). The tube comprises tiny glass fibres which can conduct light round corners so that, by looking through it once it is in place, the doctor can see into the patient's stomach.

An endoscope contains a number of channels: one with which to blow air into the stomach to distend it so that its outside edge is clearly visible; another to pump water into the stomach to wash mucus away; a third with which to remove a small piece of tissue from the stomach lining in order to perform a biopsy – an examination which would, for example, reveal the existence of any cancerous cells.

As the instrument passes down your gullet, you may feel a little discomfort and a little distension as air passes into your stomach – but nothing more than that. A lot of patients say that they cannot swallow once the endoscope is in position, but it is in fact very unusual for anyone to gag on it.

The investigation takes from two to fifteen minutes, depending on the experience of the person who is doing it. It happens sometimes, however, no matter who is doing it, that it seems to take a long time: this can be a good sign, meaning that the doctor cannot find an ulcer. He will then make a thorough search for it, appreciating that you will not want to go through the procedure again just because he did not look properly the first time. So, if it is all over within a minute of two, you would probably be right to guess that the doctor has located the offending object.

Lastly, if an ulcer is located, it may be that your doctor will wish to carry out a second endoscopy after a period of treatment to make sure that it has healed. Some experts believe, for this reason, that it is preferable to perform the investigation in the first instance under anaesthetic so that the patient does not remember what it was like. This seems slightly to conflict with claims that the patient suffers no pain during such investigations, however.

Other tests

A number of tests will be routinely carried out, particularly if you are going to have an anaesthetic: these include totally painless tests such as taking your blood pressure and blood count.

Can computers help?

Yes and no. The doctor can feed into a computer an ulcer program, when they suspect that the patient is suffering from ulceration, and this program will go through all the signs and symptoms as described at the start of this chapter. These programs will probably produce results comparable with those obtained by senior doctors, such as senior registrars and consultants. Computer programs are useful in that they remind the doctor what is important information and what is not: for example, it used to be thought the relationship between pain and food intake was important; it is now known to be less important, since half of all patients do not observe any association.

Whereas computers work in a cold, statistical and logical way, a doctor will use his or her brain to form a *general* picture of how the patient is. A computer is, in addition, fed with limited information: if a computer asks a patient about the existence of pain, the patient may be presented with options defining the extent of the pain. Where the computer fails is with the patient who responds to the doctor's question by scratching his head and saying: 'Well, yes, I do have a bit of pain.' What this actually means depends very much on the individual, how given he or she is to complaining, how nervous he or she is, what his or her pain threshold is. The statement when made by someone who has only ever been to see a doctor twice in their lives could mean something very different from the same statement made by someone who is given to headaches, insomnia, generalized anxiety attacks and frequent visits to the doctor.

Positive diagnosis

It is probably true that an experienced doctor could diagnose the presence of ulcers once he had identified the type, location, intensity and duration of the stomach pain endured by the patient, particularly if that pain is accompanied by nausea and/or vomiting. Pain causing the patient to wake during the night would confirm his suspicions and encourage him to refer the patient for immediate formal investigation, in the form either of barium X-ray or endoscopy.

Nothing is simple in medicine, but one can say that if an ulcer is detected and treated early in its life you can expect a speedy recovery to full physical health. The worst thing you can do, because you suspect that there is something moderately wrong with you, is to delay going to the doctor. By the time you are forced by the severity of the pain to visit the doctor, complications may have set in. The doctor's task is then more complex in terms of drug regime so surgery may be necessary, and your general health is more debilitated than it need have been. Provided that there are no complications, both gastric and duodenal ulcers are treated by a course of drugs these days. You stand a good chance of the ulcer healing in response to the medication and you will then have no further need of drugs. Even if complications have developed and there is a need for surgery, you may welcome this as a sign that there will eventually be an end to the nagging pain you have been enduring perhaps for months, perhaps for years.

Why me?

Ulcers are painful and inconvenient, and you may well be wondering why you have been so unlucky to develop one whereas your friend or your spouse hasn't. The next chapter looks at what the experts know so far about the type of person likely to develop an ulcer, whether they are male or female, at what age they are likely to occur and whether they run in families.

4

The Classic Ulcer Sufferer

'If you go on like this, you'll get an ulcer,' said Sally, wife of Simon, a high-flier in the marketing division of an international hotel chain. His job required him to spend a great deal of time travelling from his home in Surrey all over Europe and the United States, often at short notice, to eat in restaurants – often twice daily – and to entertain clients at presentations, cocktail parties, even at weekends: an exacting, stressful lifestyle with little provision for a healthy diet, regular sleep, exercise and relaxation. Simon represents the classic picture many of us have of the sort of person likely to develop an ulcer. This picture, however, is very much at odds with the findings of scientific research, as this chapter will show.

Stress

Stress has been held responsible for practically every medical and psychiatric condition at one time or another over the last 20 years. Only as doctors pursue their research and discover highly complex *physical* causes of many such conditions is the importance of stress being played down. Popular opinion has traditionally maintained that ulcers are produced by stress partly, perhaps, because it is known that acid is produced in the stomach in response to anger and stress, as well as to help digestion of food. And stress can, in some circumstances, produce ulcers.

Certain specific stressful situations undoubtedly do produce ulcers, but such situations are specific and usually acute. They do not include situations of a generally stressful nature such as a demanding job or bringing up a toddler and a new baby, for example, in isolation for much of the time from other adults. The best-known of these specific situations is the development of ulcers in someone who has suffered massive burns to the body or massive head injuries. It is not known why ulcers should develop after such traumas, but the evidence that they do is well substantiated.

Some years ago experiments were conducted in which rats were put under very severe stress in order to determine the role of stress in ulcers. They were made to swim for many hours in a tank out of which they could not escape. They did develop ulcers after this ordeal. However, these acute stress ulcers are different from the normal chronic ulcers that develop slowly over a long period of time and it is now thought that high-powered stressful occupations are not an important cause of ulceration.

Group exclusion

Stress sometimes affects us in unexpected ways. In the Second World War, for example, those British soldiers who were prisoners of war in German POW camps had a very low incidence of ulcers – when one might have expected them to have a high incidence. However, those same people developed ulcers much more readily when they went home to their families. As another example, during the First World War those soldiers serving at the German front seldom developed ulcers; but those waiting to go to the front much more commonly produced ulcers.

One could put forward a number of different explanations for such phenomena, including, for example, that the Second World War soldiers were not very happy with their families and the First World War men were terrified of going to the German front. However, the more plausible explanation seems to be that what is called 'group exclusion' may cause such acute (not chronic) stress as to produce ulcers. By this is meant that if you are widely supported by a network of friends and colleagues, ulceration is less likely to occur than if you are relatively isolated. This can be demonstrated by the assumption that the

Second World War soldiers took comfort in being surrounded by others in the armed forces – 'We're all in the same boat' – but felt excluded from the real business of the War when they returned home. In the case of the First World War men, it could be hypothesized that those waiting to be called up were in a somewhat dubious, even dishonourable situation; once they were at the front, they were no longer isolated and were indeed supported by the camaraderie of their peers. Both groups often experience difficulty in reintegrating themselves into life at home.

Essentially, then, it is not the pace, pressure or associated danger of your job that may produce an ulcer. What matters more is your support system and the absence of a sense of isolation. One wonders, then, if lighthouse keepers commonly develop ulcers. . .?

The sex factor

Ulcers are generally much more common in men than in women. For every three to four men with a duodenal ulcer, only one woman suffers with this problem. Gastric ulcers, too, are slightly more common in men than women. Why this is so is not known. In this century, duodenal ulcers are common and gastric ulcers are much less so, but in the nineteenth century duodenal ulcers were unknown and gastric ulcers were common, particularly so in women.

There seems so far to be no satisfactory explanation for why more men now get ulcers, nor for why the picture has changed in the last 100 years.

At what age is it likely to happen?

Although many young people get ulcers – when it is more likely to be a duodenal ulcer rather than gastric – the frequency of ulcers increases with each age group. Gastric ulcers are much more likely to develop in people over 40 than duodenal ulcers.

Women are more likely to develop ulcers after the menopause. Because of this, a possible link with the female hormone, oestrogen, produced as part of the menstrual cycle, has been considered, but there is no conclusive evidence pointing to the presence of oestrogen playing a protective role.

In general, ulcers are much more common in middle-aged and elderly people: it is not a young person's disease.

Does it run in families?

Some families have a definite history of developing ulcers but they are unusual. Ulcers *can* run in families, but the association is not a strong one. If a close relative of yours has an ulcer, you are a little more likely to develop one yourself, but by no means certain to do so.

Ulcers are not hereditary in the sense that a particular gene is responsible for them, as is the case, for example, in muscular dystrophy, Huntington's chorea and schizophrenia. Like many common diseases, peptic ulcer disease is caused by a confusing mix of genetic and environmental factors.

Natural tendencies

Your genetic make-up has some further bearing on whether or not you develop an ulcer. For example, you are slightly more likely to get an ulcer if your blood is group O than if it is group A, B or AB. There could be a link here with the fact that people with blood group O are also more likely to develop the complication of bleeding from their ulcers. If you have a bleeding ulcer, this serious condition is unlikely to be over-looked by a doctor; if, however, the ulcer is not bleeding and you happen to have an irregular indigestion, a doctor may not notice that you have an ulcer, unless you have a full hospital investigation as described in Chapter 3. So, it could be that it is not so much that those with blood group O get more ulcers but that they are more efficiently diagnosed because theirs tend more commonly to bleed.

There is another aspect to your body's make-up which may have a bearing on whether you are likely to get an ulcer. All of us have glycoproteins, which are complex molecules that determine what our blood group is. Most people secrete these substances into the saliva and into the gastric mucus, the sticky stuff that lines and protects the gut. These people are less likely to develop ulcers. About one in five people, however, known as non-secretors, do not secrete glycoproteins into the saliva and they are more likely to get an ulcer. One in three ulcer patients is a non-secretor.

Where you live

The rate of ulcer sufferers tends to be higher in urban areas than in rural areas, but not much higher. City life cannot be held responsible for your ulcer, however, although it could be a contributing factor.

It has been established that you are less likely to develop an ulcer if you live in the South of England than the North, irrespective of whether you live in a city. One large study compared hospital inpatients from Leeds, Newcastle, Manchester and Liverpool with patients from London, Oxford, Wessex and the South-West. It was found that those patients from the northern cities suffered in greater numbers in almost all classifications – non-perforated and perforated duodenal ulcer and non-perforated and perforated gastric ulcer. The reasons for this picture are undoubtedly complex and as yet unresolved.

It is also known that people living in Scotland are more prone to develop ulcers than those living in England. The distribution is similarly uneven in Europe with big variations from one country to another. Why this is so is not understood; these days one might quickly suspect a poor diet as the culprit but there is simply no evidence to support this idea.

If you happen to live in Southern India, where rice is the staple, you are much more likely to develop an ulcer than if you live in the North, where wheat would be your staple. The wheat is unprocessed and such a diet is classified therefore as a high masticatory diet and high in fibre. Again, one might assume that diet holds the key with foods rich in fibre as the answer. However, it has not been possible to prove this. The only piece of evidence to support this idea emerged in 1982 when it was shown that a low intake of fibre diminishes duodenal ulcer healing: and this is not the same as stating that high-fibre diets prevent ulcers.

Is diet important?

Doctors have traditionally not been over concerned with diet and are not trained in nutrition. One may assume, therefore, that their research studies are unlikely to take them down this path. The long-suffering ulcer patient in the 1960s was exhorted to eat plain white fish. If they did not get better, they were asked which method of cooking they had used – if they had steamed the fish they were told to boil it, and if they had boiled it they were told to steam it!

To date high-fibre diets have been researched and scientifically investigated and it has proved impossible to show that lots of bran will prevent you developing an ulcer. Low-carbohydrate diets have also been looked at but, again, the results have been inconclusive. (It was thought that there might be a link between a high carbohydrate content in the stomach with excessive acid secretion.)

Other theories have suggested that lots of vitamin C and fresh vegetables are important in preventing ulcers, but this still remains controversial.

Although a lot of research has gone on into different diets and no clear and consistent pattern has emerged, some experts are still left with a lingering suspicion that the people of northern India who eat lots of wheat, in the form of chapattis, and have to chew a great deal, may in some way be protecting themselves from developing an ulcer.

Drinking

Surprisingly, alcohol no longer appears to be an important determining factor of whether or not you get ulcers. However, most experts would agree that you should not imbibe alcohol on an empty stomach, nor should you take a drink during an attack of pain.

Both coffee and cola drinks are known to be bad for ulcer patients. Their common ingredient is caffeine which is known to stimulate acid secretion in the stomach. Because of the increased acid in the stomach, it is not surprising that both coffee and cola drinkers suffer more with ulcers. What is perhaps surprising is that even two cups of coffee per day *doubles* the risk of getting an ulcer compared with those people who don't drink anything containing caffeine at all. Curiously, some experts claim that coffee is harmful in this context, irrespective of whether it contains caffeine or not, so they would assert that decaffeinated coffee will not protect you from the possibility of developing an ulcer.

The best bet for the ulcer sufferer is fresh milk because it is an antacid, and therefore helps to counteract the action of stomach acids.

Does my job make a difference?

Social class and occupation do show consistent patterns among those who develop ulcers. It used to be thought a rather upper-class thing to have a duodenal ulcer, but it is now known that this is a misconception. Social class D, which comprises unskilled workers and manual labourers, has a much higher incidence of ulcers than social class A, which includes, for example, doctors and lawyers.

A clue to why this should be lies in the fact that those in social class D smoke more, and it is smokers who are more likely to develop ulcers. Even when the smoking factor is taken into account, however, social class D still shows a higher rate of ulcers. It is not known why this should be, but it is possible that diet and blood group could play a part.

'No thanks, I don't smoke'

There is no doubt that smokers fare badly in terms of ulceration and, indeed, with many other diseases. They respond less well to treatment, they are more likely to have ulcers and they are more likely to have complications.

Unfortunately for light smokers, it does not appear to matter very much how much you smoke or whether or not you have given up smoking. The risk remains. Even if you were a smoker twenty years ago, your chances of getting an ulcer appear to be *double* those of people who have never smoked.

The damage caused to the body by smoking is important in the cause of ulcers. In addition, however, some experts believe that there is a link between those people who show a predisposition to ulcer disease and those who become addicted to smoking. This is not the same as saying that smoking *causes* ulcers, although smoking is undoubtedly an important factor in the cause.

'And now this, too'

Some people get ulcers simply because they are taking drugs for another condition and those other drugs actually cause ulceration of the lining of the gut. Unfortunately, some of those conditions are so serious that these people cannot simply stop taking the drugs.

There is some controversy about how important the various anti-arthritic drugs, for example, are in causing ulcers. Some experts believe that this is rare. Most of the arthritic drugs, including aspirin, work as prostaglandin inhibitors. Prostaglandin is important in improving the protection of the stomach and therefore diminishing the effect of the acid upon the lining of the stomach. Because prostaglandin plays this important role, it is not surprising that anti-arthritic drugs, which inhibit prostaglandin, may allow the stomach wall to become weakened and allow ulcers to develop or recur.

During a hospital investigation, when a doctor places an aspirin on the surface of the patient's stomach, he can see a little later, with the help of an endoscope, a small haemorrhage on the stomach wall where the aspirin has done some damage. It is difficult, nevertheless, to provide hard evidence that aspirin takers are more at risk from developing ulcers than others.

For some reason, which is not fully understood, Australians tend to consume very large amounts of aspirin. There is evidence to show that the heaviest consumers are more likely to get ulcers. However, the average person who may take one or two aspirins a day or a week is not really any more likely to get ulcers.

The main controversy at the moment really surrounds whether elderly people, who are the commonest group taking anti-arthritic drugs on a regular basis, are more likely to get ulcers which are more likely to perforate or bleed. Some English studies suggest that this is the case, but recent American studies have dismissed the idea.

Many people have such bad pain in their joints that they must take effective drugs for their arthritis and they may therefore have to take the slightly increased risk of ulcers as well as a perforation and bleeding. However, such people should be made aware that if the drugs for the relief of the arthritis do not seem to be doing much good, they should turn to a simpler painkiller, such as paracetamol, which has never been shown to damage the stomach and would do just as well.

If you already have attacks of ulcer pain and you require an anti-arthritic pill, your doctor is often in a considerable dilemma. He will tend to give you an ulcer-healing drug, such as cimetidine (see Chapter 5), coupled with your arthritis medication. Although many doctors believe that this does some good, there is no actual evidence to support the belief.

Certainly, if you have indigestion and you are not sure whether your anti-arthritis pills are doing you any good, it is well worth stopping them for a period, seeing if the indigestion improves, and trying instead simple painkillers, such as paracetamol which do not damage the stomach.

Another group of drugs that may cause ulcers are steroids. Again, doctors are not in total agreement about this: it is not known whether people on steroids are more inclined to have ulcers because of the disease from which they suffer, necessitating the steroids, or because of the steroid treatment itself.

There is also some doubt about whether steroids make ulcers more likely to perforate. Steroids are given to reduce the degree of inflammation and fibrosis (the formation of scar tissue) that certain diseases produce; when fibrosis is inhibited, an ulcer can develop deeper into the stomach wall, because it is prevented from healing itself naturally and forming scar tissue. It may then continue and perforate.

More people take steroids for very serious conditions and could not possibly stop without consulting their doctor. The importance of the underlying condition for which the steroids are given is usually such that it is not possible to change the dose. Such people with indigestion or ulcers who have to take steroids should be offered other ulcer healing drugs in order to try and reduce the risk of complications.

An overall picture

It is clear, then, from modern research that the traditional picture of an ulcer sufferer is far removed from the truth. The man with ulcers will probably be at least middle aged, his father may have had ulcers, he will perhaps live in Scotland, he may eat a lot of pappy food that does not need much chewing, he may not be a muesli addict, he may be a manual labourer, his blood group may be O and he will probably be a smoker. It is more likely, however, that he will exhibit some of these characteristics rather than all of them. Your friend with ulcers may be a middle-aged woman who lives in Surrey, is bored and isolated, smokes and drinks coffee a lot and takes a lot of aspirin for headaches.

5

Treating Ulcers

The treatment of ulcers has altered very dramatically in the last
20 years or so. Patients used to be told to stick to a bland diet of
steamed white fish and not to exert themselves. They were also
operated on very much more frequently than is the case these
days – there are now a number of drugs on the market that, if
taken regularly, can heal ulcers without the need for a stay in
hospital.

Duodenal ulcers tend to respond better to drugs than gastric
ulcers. Some patients with gastric ulcers get better as a result of
a course of drugs, but some find that the problem recurs a few
months later. There is an additional problem with gastric
ulcers, in that they could be gastric cancers rather than ulcers,
and for this reason an endoscopic investigation (described in
Chapter 3), before accepting prescription drugs for this
condition, is a must. This problem is discussed more fully at the
end of this chapter.

Ulcer complications – bleeding, haemorrhage, perforation,
pyloric stenosis – cannot be cured with drugs and will require an
operation as soon as possible. Because of this risk of complications, you are urged, if you have the typical symptoms of an
ulcer sufferer (see Chapter 3) to consult a doctor without delay.

Treatment for ulcers falls into two main categories – drugs
and surgery, of which the first is nowadays the most common. In
order to understand better why you have been prescribed a
certain drug, you need to know a bit about how it works and
what causes your ulcer (see Chapter 2). Drug treatments fall
into two categories: those that are intended to control the
amount of acid that is produced in your stomach, one of the key
factors in the development of ulcers, and those that strengthen
your stomach lining so that it is better able to withstand the
onslaught of your acid secretions. This chapter discusses not

only those drugs commonly used today to heal ulcers, but also those that have been frequently used in the past, as some people will still be taking them.

Before we look at what sort of over-the-counter and prescription drugs and surgical techniques are available to you, it is worth looking briefly at what your lifestyle can do for you in terms of treatment, notably in your diet and whether or not you are a smoker. These things are important factors in your treatment, but they will also be discussed more fully in later chapters.

What should I eat?

In the days when doctors had no effective treatment for ulcers, they were very keen to try and explain to the patient that diet was important. We are all aware that certain foods upset us and this is obviously true of people with peptic ulcers; such people should avoid food that seems consistently to cause more pain. However, some ulcer patients are perfectly happy eating curries and drinking alcohol and this does not seem to be any worse or better for them than eating steamed fish. Much of the talk about diet in ulcers is rubbish. It is known that taking small, frequent meals will reduce the pain of an ulcer, but what is really important is early and effective treatment.

Smoking

It is important to try and give up smoking as most drugs, with the exception of De Nol (described in Part Two of this chapter), work less effectively in smokers who, besides having their ulcers for longer, also seem more likely to develop serious complications (see Chapter 2).

PART 1: REDUCING THE ACID IN YOUR STOMACH

Antacids and milk

Some drugs and treatments can be used to relieve symptoms and others can also be used to heal ulcers. During the course of healing, of course, the ulcer pain improves. Eating foods, or taking antacids (such as Rennies or Milk of Magnesia) or milk may relieve some of your symptoms, particularly pain. Antacids have an odd effect on pain in ulcers because they work very quickly, long before you'd expect the buffering capacity to influence the degree of acidity in the stomach. As well as this, the strength of the antacid doesn't seem to be related to its efficiency in inhibiting the pain. So, you should choose any antacid which suits you. There are also a number of different tablets, available both over-the-counter and on prescription, which work in essentially the same way.

Those that contain magnesium tend to produce diarrhoea, while those that contain aluminium tend to produce constipation. Treatments that contain a mixture of the two, such as Maalox, may enable the constipation and diarrhoea to counteract each other so that the bowel motion is relatively normal.

If you have heart problems, you should try and avoid those antacids that contain a lot of sodium. Years ago a problem with raised calcium levels in the bloodstream occurred if you took too much milk, together with antacids that contained a lot of calcium, or other alkali compounds. This was called the milk-alkali syndrome. Now that there are much more effective remedies for treating ulcers, fortunately, most people don't take antacids in such large quantities.

Anticholinergic drugs

Acid secretion in the stomach starts as soon as we smell or taste food. The secretion is controlled by one of the parasympathetic nerves, the *vagus* nerve. The acid itself is stimulated by a chemical called acetylcholine which is delivered from the nerve endings into the stomach. It is possible to inhibit or reduce the effect of the acetylcholine with anticholinergic substances: these inhibit the amount of acid produced in the stomach and thus give your ulcer a chance to heal.

Anticholinergic drugs, such as probanthine, for example, were once widely used but they tend to be less so now, partly because of the side-effects they cause and partly because there are now better drugs on the market. Side-effects were caused by the drug inhibiting the action of acetylcholine not only in the stomach but also in the rest of the body. This meant that you might suffer with a dry mouth, or find it difficult to focus your eyes properly. This could be dangerous if you also had glaucoma. Some patients also experience difficulty in passing urine; and this is particularly severe in men if the prostate is already enlarged. This is a common condition in older men, in whom ulcers are in any case more common than in women.

H_2 antagonists

Acid is also produced in the stomach by another chemical, known as histamine, which acts directly on the cells of the stomach to make it produce acid. Histamine produces a variety of symptoms in different parts of the body – nettle rash, for example – and these can usually be controlled with drugs called antihistamines. It long puzzled medical scientists, however, that the well-known antihistamines, such as Triludan, failed to have any effect on acid secretion in the stomach. Eventually it was realized that the system in the stomach which responds to histamine – the 'receptor' – is different from the system in other parts of the body, so ordinary antihistamines couldn't affect it. To overcome this, a new kind of antihistamine was developed. These are known as H_2 antagonists, which simply means that they work on this second type of histamine receptor. They inhibit the action of histamine on the stomach, and thus also inhibit acid production. The appearance of H_2 antagonists, such as cimetidine, was the beginning of the breakthrough that led to such effective treatment for ulcers.

Gastrin

The third means by which acid is produced in the stomach is by means of a hormone called *gastrin*. This hormone is secreted at the lower end of the stomach when food stimulates it and this therefore turns the acid secretion on in the stomach at the time when it is needed, that is, when we've just eaten. Doctors have not yet found a way to inhibit gastrin-induced acid secretion with medicines, but this is one of the ways in which surgery works (described in Part Three of this chapter). Surgery removes the gastrin-secreting part of the stomach and so when we eat food there is no extra stimulus to acid production.

Are they effective?

If we can keep the acid concentration in the stomach down consistently throughout the day, then ulcers will heal and any agent which will effectively reduce acid secretion will work in healing ulcers equally effectively. The anticholinergic drugs that have already been mentioned, if given in high doses continuously, will suppress acid secretion sufficiently to allow ulcers to heal, but, as previously mentioned, the side-effects of these drugs means that these agents are not now widely used. In the same way, large doses of antacids taken every few hours will also allow ulcers to heal. However, the standard dose of Maalox, for example, to allow this to happen (30 ml five times a day) means that you often get bowel problems and also that you have to carry large amounts of antacids around with you and remember to take them on a frequent basis. Research shows that, while some Americans are apparently prepared to do this, most Europeans find this process very inconvenient.

Cimetidine

The first effective H_2 antagonist was cimetidine, now a very widely used drug. This drug has now been given to many millions of people over at least the last 15 years in many countries of the world and is one of the safest drugs on the market.

Because ulcers will often heal spontaneously of their own accord, if sufficient time is allowed, it was therefore important for doctors to be certain that H_2 antagonists were *more* effective than the body's natural ability to heal ulcers itself: the original research studies of cimetidine were all done by what are called placebo-controlled trials. This means that neither the patient, nor the doctor, knew whether the patient was taking an active drug or a placebo (which looked the same but contained nothing more than chalk). The patients were all known to have ulcers before the study started because they had been examined with an endoscope (see Chapter 3); whether or not the ulcer had healed was determined by a second endoscopy six weeks after the start of treatment.

Many studies of this sort have now been done and it has been shown that about 40 per cent of all duodenal ulcers heal with a placebo after six weeks (natural and spontaneous healing in other words), whereas 80–90 per cent of all patients treated with cimetidine will heal. Gastric ulcers do not heal quite as well as duodenal ulcers and some 70 per cent of patients with duodenal ulcers will heal after six weeks, compared with up to 50 per cent of those treated with a placebo.

Cimetidine was proved to be an effective agent for both types of ulcers, therefore, but more so for duodenal ulcers. There are many reasons why ulcers may not heal within a six-week period. First, the ulcer may be very large and therefore take longer to heal. Second, many patients stop taking their medicine, unfortunately, as soon as their pain is relieved – if the ulcer has not healed, continuing to take the tablets regularly is essential. Finally, patients who continue to smoke while taking the tablets find that their ulcers heal less effectively and less quickly. There is also probably a small core of patients who for some reason are resistant to H_2 antagonists and do not heal whatever dose is given.

When should I take it?

Initially, cimetidine was given four times a day because it was thought to be very important to stop acid production throughout the day. However, it is now realized that the most important time to stop acid production is during the night and therefore taking cimetidine in a dose of 800 mg at night is probably just as good a way as taking the tablets several times throughout the day. This is obviously much easier as you don't have to carry the drugs around with you.

Is it safe?

Cimetidine is a very safe drug, but there are a few very rare side-effects. The trouble with all drugs is that when some patients are given tablets they tend to assume that any symptoms are due to the tablet on which they are placed. Many people given placebo tablets, such as chalk, for example, complain of a large number of side-effects, particularly nausea, headache, vomiting, dizziness, etc. Nevertheless, over the years, it has been realized that there are a few genuine side-effects of cimetidine which are commoner in patients who take the active drug than those taking a placebo. The important ones are that old people occasionally become confused, that a few people get palpitations and irregular heart rhythms and that, very occasionally, cimetidine has an inhibiting effect on the normal male hormones. Men may develop small breasts and become impotent. Fortunately, this is usually reversible when the drug is stopped.

Cimetidine may also stimulate the liver enzymes which normally process other drugs in the body. These drugs may be less effective, therefore, when taken with cimetidine. This is not an important problem providing that the doctor remembers, or you remind him, that you are taking cimetidine as well as other drugs (for example, blood-thinning drugs, such as Warfarin, or anti-epileptic drugs such as phenytoin), so that he or she adjusts the dose accordingly.

Ranitidine

A newer agent which is also now being very widely used is called ranitidine or Zantac. This drug is just as effective as cimetidine and appears to have none of cimetidine's side-effects. This is obviously a great advantage and one would expect to find it in as widespread use as cimetidine. However, because cimetidine has been around so long and because doctors are always worried that a very unusual side-effect of a drug will occur many years after its introduction, cimetidine is often prescribed in preference.

You should be aware that things can just rarely go wrong: a drug called Practolol, for example, quite unexpectedly produced damage to the intestines many years after its first introduction. To try and avoid this complication with the new anti-ulcer drugs, very careful surveillance of all patients taking the drugs is now maintained, so that any possible side-effects can be rapidly announced. Fortunately, both cimetidine and ranitidine have been so widely used that the possibility that an unusual side-effect will occur in the future is now very slight.

What's new?

A very new drug called omeprazole is just being introduced in some countries. This drug also inhibits acid, but in a different way from the H_2 antagonists. This is a very strong compound which can inhibit acid production completely. It probably does not have any advantages over the already widely used drugs for most patients with ulcers, but it may be more effective for the small number of patients who don't heal with the normal H_2 antagonists. It may also prove to be a good drug to treat heartburn (described in Chapter 1) where complete inhibition of acid may be very important.

There is absolutely no evidence that any of the H_2 antagonists make you more likely to develop cancer of the stomach, although this is something that receives a lot of publicity from the Press. These worries may be a little more firmly founded in the case of omeprazole for two reasons: first, omeprazole is a very powerful inhibiter of acid, and second, because it is believed that the presence of *some* stomach acid protects against the development of gastric cancer. Many experts believe that gastric cancer is partially produced by bacteria, which can grow in the stomach in the absence of any acid; these bacteria are killed if there is plenty of acid remaining in the stomach. It is unlikely, therefore, that you would be prescribed omeprazole for longer than a six-week course.

For how long should I take the drugs?

One of the disappointments with the treatment of ulcers in the past was that, although one could heal most of them within six weeks on taking an H_2 antagonist, the ulcer often recurred quite rapidly. The drugs failed to prevent the periodic comings and goings of pain, which have been discussed in Chapter 3.

There are two ways round this problem. It is quite possible to take the H_2 antagonists continuously for long periods, usually taking one tablet nightly. This means that the number of ulcers causing symptoms is very small and that the patient is pain-free most of the time. However, despite taking drugs continuously, perhaps one in three patients examined with an endoscope will be found to have an ulcer, even though it is producing no symptoms. It is not known whether these ulcers which are producing no symptoms are still likely to perforate or bleed. If continuous medication were to prevent these complications, many doctors might advise most patients to have this sort of treatment. However, what most doctors advise is to take a course of tablets and then stop. About half the patients will have no further trouble for a year, but the other half will again get typical ulcer pain within a few months. If this happens to you, you will probably recognize very rapidly what the pain is due to on the second occasion and should in any case go to the doctor for further treatment.

If the first ulcer was a duodenal ulcer, your doctor will usually be willing to give further treatment without any additional investigations as most people get ulcers in the same place on the second occasion and these usually respond to a further course of treatment. If the ulcer was a gastric ulcer, there is a very small risk that this is actually an ulcerating cancer, discussed more fully at the end of this chapter, and most doctors will want to be sure, therefore, on each occasion that the pain occurs, that the ulcer in the stomach is benign and that there is no evidence of cancer.

This recurrent use of drugs whenever the pain returns works well for many patients. However, if you are having three or four attacks of pain every year, it is probably better to take the drugs every night and so prevent most of the pain altogether. Taking H_2 antagonists, such as cimetidine, continuously for many years is safe and there are now many millions of patients all over the world who have taken the drugs with no adverse side-effects.

What are the alternatives?

Anti-depressants have been tried from time to time to heal ulcers and do so quite successfully. Many people believed that this was because stress tended to produce more ulcers. We now know that this is probably not the case in general (see Chapter 4), but anti-depressants nevertheless remain an effective ulcer healing agent. This is probably because most anti-depressants are also anti-cholinergic agents; in other words, they stop the reaction of the vagus nerve which controls acid secretion in the stomach.

There are some other agents which your doctor may give you which are also effective at healing your ulcer. One is famotidine, which is another H_2 antagonist, but which doesn't seem to have any particular advantages over the well-known substances. Another is gastrozepin, an anticholinergic agent, which doesn't seem to have many of the side-effects of the other anticholinergic drugs and so most patients are happy to take it. Again, there don't appear to be any significant advantages over the other compounds that have been mentioned.

PART 2: STRENGTHENING THE STOMACH

It was noted at the start of this chapter that the strength of the lining of the stomach and the gut is as important as the effect of the acid upon that lining. Another way to heal ulcers, therefore, is not to worry about the acid but instead to strengthen the normal protective mechanisms of the stomach. As you will have read in Chapter 2, these are concerned both with the mucus and the cell lining of the stomach. Some drugs, such as De Nol, do this. De Nol was known about long before cimetidine was introduced, but because it has a rather unpleasant taste and also contains bismuth, which may be toxic if taken for long periods, it was never widely prescribed. In fact, De Nol is just as effective at inhibiting ulcers as any of the H_2 antagonists. It is a horrid-smelling liquid that has to be taken five times a day. The smell of the liquid and its taste can be improved by allowing it to stand in the air for five minutes before drinking it down, but the situation has recently been much improved by the introduction of tablets which are easy to swallow without all the problems of taste.

The case for De Nol

De Nol is a valuable drug because it is one of the few that seem to be able to reduce the likelihood of your ulcer returning. If after a six-week course of cimetidine, 100 patients are monitored for a year, 90 will have had a recurrent ulcer as shown by endoscopic investigation within that year. However, if De Nol is given for six weeks to heal the ulcer, then only 40 to 50 will have a recurrent ulcer within the year. In addition, De Nol appears to heal ulcers in smokers as effectively as in those who don't smoke, and De Nol may also work in the small hard core of patients who don't get better with the H_2 antagonists.

All these facts mean that De Nol is being increasingly used in the treatment of ulcers. It is not used more because it is foul to take and because it contains bismuth. Although bismuth in the form of De Nol has never been shown to have any toxic effects, there is always a worry that this metal may cause damage to the brain or to the kidneys if used long-term, and so the licence allowing De Nol to be used does not allow it to be used for more than six weeks at a time.

Another exciting fact about De Nol is its effect on a bacterium called *campylobacter pyloridis*. This bug is present in a very high proportion of patients who have an ulcer and some experts believe that this is the most important reason that ulcers occur. How this organism causes ulcers is not clear and how it gets into the body is also not clear. However, De Nol appears to be able to kill these bacteria whereas cimetidine cannot. If this is eventually proved to be the case, it will explain why De Nol appears to be effective long after a patient has stopped taking it, whereas the effect of cimetidine is lost within a few days of stopping the drug.

The alternatives to De Nol

Another drug that strengthens the stomach's mucosal layer is sucralphate. This is a complex aluminium compound which works just as effectively as cimetidine or De Nol. It is widely used in some countries, but less so in the United Kingdom.

The original mucosal protective agent and the first drug ever shown to heal ulcers was a drug called carbenoxolone, a pure substance extracted from the root of liquorice plant. This drug has an interesting history. It was noticed in the 1940s that the Dutch had a very low incidence of ulcers during the Second World War and in 1946 it was decided to try and find out why. It was known that the Dutch were very short of food during the War and that they used to eat sticks of liquorice from the fields. It was decided, therefore, to find out if there was an active compound in liquorice which helped ulcers to heal. This turned out to be carbenoxolone sodium and many studies were done by eminent gastroenterologists which showed that this would increase the rapidity with which gastric ulcers healed.

Unfortunately, particularly in old people, carbenoxolone may have two serious side-effects. One is a loss of potassium from the body, which makes you feel very weak, and the other is retention of sodium in the body. This is normally excreted in the kidneys; if it is not, it can cause heart failure and also cause the ankles to swell. For this reason this drug is very little used now, although it is probably safe in young people. One elderly patient who was kept on carbenoxolone sodium for a year did not have her potassium level checked at all. At this point she had not been out of the house for nine months: she was completely bedridden. She had been told that this was because she had a cancerous growth of the ovary which was untreatable. Fortunately, an excellent consultant physician at another hospital had her potassium level checked and found it was only a quarter of normal. She was given extra potassium and she got off her bed and walked – a true miracle, as it seemed to the patient.

Various derivatives of liquorice, which don't cause these side-effects, have been developed. The most widely used of these is a compound called Caved/S. This appears to be effective in healing ulcers without many side-effects, but it's never been very popular.

New developments

There is a special chemical in the blood called *prostaglandin* which may be very important in keeping the mucosal barrier of the stomach strong. Various chemicals similar to prosta-glandins are now under investigation to see if they can replicate the role of the natural substance. These can certainly strength-en the mucosal barrier of the stomach and also inhibit gastric acid. In some ways, this might seem an ideal combination, but in big research studies these substances (methyl-substituted prostaglandins) are no more effective than the drugs presently available, and in addition, unfortunately, they cause a little

61

diarrhoea and they *might* induce abortion in women who are in early pregnancy. Although this latter side-effect is unlikely and the first one is not serious, it has meant that the licensing authorities have so far not allowed this substance to come on to the market.

PART 3: THE CASE FOR AN OPERATION

The use of very effective drugs to heal ulcers has obviously caused a great reduction in the number of surgical operations. Some people, however, are unwilling to take tablets for too long and would rather have an operation than continue with medication. Other people with one of the three major complications of ulcers (bleeding, perforation and pyloric stenosis) will need an operation anyway.

There are a number of operations that can be performed, and they are all designed to reduce the amount of acid secretion in the stomach. The three main ones are:

partial gastrectomy; vagotomy combined with pyloroplasty; and highly selective vagotomy.

The most effective of these, the partial gastrectomy, involves cutting away a large portion of the stomach. This both removes the total capacity of the stomach to produce acid, and, even more importantly, reduces the size of the lower part of the stomach called the *antrum*, which is the part with the most gastrin, one of the hormones that stimulates acid secretion. Although this operation is the most effective at preventing ulcers from recurring, it is also the operation involving the highest risk of death and the operation with the most side-effects.

Vagotomy combined with pyloroplasty involves cutting the main nerve to the stomach, the vagus, in order to reduce the amount of acid secretion. The vagus is also important in allowing the stomach to drain properly, and so, if the vagus alone is cut, food cannot leave the stomach. So, in addition to cutting the vagus, an operation to allow the stomach to drain more easily, by making a bigger hole at the end of the stomach (the pylorus), is also performed.

Vagotomy and pyloroplasty is a safer operation than partial gastrectomy, but unfortunately the rate of ulcers returning, despite the operation, is about one in ten. There are also quite a lot of side-effects from this operation. It is believed that most of these side-effects are due to the drainage procedure and the fact that the main vagus nerve supplies not only the stomach, but all the rest of the bowel as well.

A different operation has therefore been devised in which just the nerves coming off the vagus which go to the stomach are divided, but the nerve to the pylorus is left intact. This is called a 'highly selective' vagotomy and means that there is no drainage procedure required of the stomach. Certainly, the side-effects from this operation are few, but the rate of recurrence is even higher, perhaps one in seven.

What are the side-effects?

The side-effects of all these operations are, firstly, that the patient may feel full after a small meal and therefore tend to lose some weight, which if you are underweight or elderly may not be a good thing. Second, the normal propulsion of the intestines is reduced and bugs which do not normally grow in the small intestine flourish and produce diarrhoea. This is rare with highly selective vagotomy, but common when the main vagus itself is divided. This diarrhoea is usually just a nuisance, but occasionally it can be very severe, leading to incontinence and to the patient's becoming a recluse and having to live near a lavatory. This is sometimes a problem every day, but sometimes it occurs in bouts which last for only a few days at a time. In addition to these side-effects, the patient often becomes anaemic in later years because he or she cannot absorb iron properly and, more rarely, they cannot absorb other vitamins, particularly B_{12} (the factor that prevents pernicious anaemia) and folic acid. All patients who have had a stomach operation should take a course of iron tablets every year to boost their iron stores and some will require injections of vitamin B_{12} after several years.

Another side-effect is that, occasionally, the absorption of calcium from the body is not normal and the bones become demineralized, giving rise to osteoporosis and back pain. In addition to this rare side-effect, there is a worry that many years after a partial gastrectomy, the chances of having cancer of the stomach may be increased. Indeed, recent studies have shown that the chances of having cancer anywhere in the body are increased, perhaps because the stomach now allows the toxins that cause cancer into the body; these would have been destroyed previously by the acid of the stomach.

It should be emphasized that these side-effects are not common and should not put you off having an operation if you really need it.

Essential surgery

One of the circumstances in which an operation is obviously necessary is if you are bleeding heavily. Most commonly the bleeding stops and the patient can be treated with a blood transfusion and H_2 antagonists. Occasionally, however, after a day or so of the bleeding being stopped, the bleeding restarts and occasionally the bleeding does not stop at all. In both of these circumstances an operation is necessary. The simplest operation is simply to sew up the artery lying within the ulcer that is causing the bleeding and then for the patient to take a course of drugs. However, many doctors believe that while the surgeon is operating, it is sensible to try and prevent the ulcer from recurring by doing one of the operations described above.

If you are unlucky enough to have an ulcer which perforates

the lining of the gut, the stomach contents pass into the abdominal cavity. This is a medical emergency which always requires an emergency operation. The operation is quite straightforward and simply involves sewing the hole up. Again, if the surgeon is experienced, he may well want to prevent the ulcer from recurring by doing an operation that will prevent this in the future, as discussed above.

Pyloric stenosis is a condition in which the patient continues to vomit old food. Again, there is no medicine that will work here and the patient will need an operation so that the stomach can be drained through a separate hole into the small intestine. The ulcers which usually cause pyloric stenosis are close to the exit of the stomach, that is, in the duodenum or in the pylorus.

Will it hurt?

Most stomach operations are fairly straightforward and would mean a stay in hospital of about ten days. For the first few days after an operation, the stomach does not work properly and therefore a tube drains the stomach contents through the nose to the outside. This nasogastric tube is uncomfortable, but you will probably be fairly sleepy throughout most of the first two or three days after the operation. The wound is also painful and this is a particular problem because, after any operation of this sort, it is important to keep the lungs moving well and so the physiotherapist will come round and expect you to do deep breathing exercises and move about – and this is all the more difficult to do because of the pain of the operation scar.

In the future

One of the most exciting recent advances in medicine for ulcer patients is the use of lasers to stop ulcers bleeding. When examining a patient who is bleeding, the doctor can sometimes see, with the help of an endoscope, the blood spurting out of the base of an ulcer; and it is sometimes possible to see the blood vessel or artery which has a hole in it. Scientific developments have allowed a very thin laser beam to be passed through the endoscope and this can fry the bleeding vessel and so stop the patient from bleeding to death. This procedure is still in its experimental stages, however, and it is not yet known whether this treatment will help those who are bleeding massively and who would otherwise require an operation.

Special problems with gastric ulcers

Gastric ulcers are somewhat less likely than duodenal ulcers to heal with the available drugs, as was said at the start of this chapter. The additional problem is that about 10 per cent of patients who appear to have gastric ulcers in fact have a gastric cancer. People with ordinary gastric ulcers will probably not develop gastric cancers within ulcers, but about one in ten people who have what looks like, on a barium X-ray, a simple gastric ulcer, in fact has a gastric cancer, even though they have the symptoms of an ulcer. For these reasons, all people with gastric ulcers should have an endoscopy (see Chapter 3). The doctor can then look at the ulcer carefully, when it may be obvious that it is a cancer, rather than a simple ulcer. Sometimes, however, the distinction, even with an endoscopic investigation, is not clear. In such cases the doctor will take a little bit of tissue from the ulcer and look at it under a microscope (a biopsy). He can be certain in this way whether or not it is a benign simple ulcer, or in fact a gastric cancer.

Because there is room for confusion in diagnosis, doctors should be reluctant to give patients ulcer treatment simply on the basis of their symptoms. These gastric ulcer cancers will often get better for a time on H_2 antagonists or other treatment and the patient (and the doctor) is therefore lulled into a false sense of security. This risk is *very low* below the age of 50 and some doctors believe that it is perfectly safe to give people with typical symptoms treatment for their ulcer without further investigation. However, all doctors would probably accept that it is very important to be sure that all patients over the age of 50 have at least a barium meal or an endoscopy to exclude a gastric ulcer as a cause of the symptoms.

Will the treatment work?

This question has been answered to some extent in this chapter and will be discussed more fully in Chapters 6 and 7. One of the themes to emerge is the importance of taking the drugs that have been prescribed for you at the right time of day and in the correct dosage. This at least is up to you and it is worth noting here that you can take some responsibility for your return to good health: always check with the doctor, when you actually see him or her, what the drug is, what the dosage is and when you are meant to take the medication. All human beings are fallible, and it is not uncommon therefore for the doctor to write out the prescription incorrectly or for the chemist to make it up wrongly. When you receive the made-up prescription, check the label and make sure that it tallies with what the doctor told you in his consulting room.

Lastly, do remember that it is essential for you to take the tablets for the full course – don't stop taking them as soon as the pain has stopped because the ulcer will not yet be fully healed and may, therefore, recur.

6

What if it Doesn't Get Better?

Whether or not you recover completely from your ulcer depends partly on what caused it, partly on your own disposition to developing ulcers and partly upon the treatment selected to heal it. The different types of treatment, notably drugs and surgery, are discussed in full in Chapter 5, together with the likely outcome of these treatments. Most treatments have one side-effect or another and it is also unfortunately the case that some people will relapse with another ulcer. Some people, however, heal completely and have no further problems. It is also known that ulcers can heal of their own accord with neither drug treatments nor surgery, provided that you are in good general health.

Getting better

Many years ago, before the existence of good drug treatments for ulcers, a South London GP called Dr Fry looked at what happened to those of his patients who developed ulcer pain. He found that in the majority of patients the pain had subsided completely, with no further relapses, by ten years. At most, some patients experienced attacks of pain for four or five years and they then healed.

This is fairly reassuring in that it seems that ulcer disease is not necessarily a lifelong condition. It should be remembered, however, that Dr Fry was a general practitioner not a hospital doctor. He would have seen patients, therefore, whose condition was not so bad that they needed to be treated as a hospital inpatient or outpatient. It has to be assumed that Dr Fry's worst cases, and indeed those of any GP, are sent to hospital, where the picture is rather different.

Fewer operations

A fair proportion of those who are supervised with hospital treatment carry on having ulcer symptoms for many years and end up having an operation. The situation has been radically changed by the introduction of good drugs and now it is the case that far fewer operations for peptic ulcers are performed.

Initially, when the H_2 antagonists (see Chapter 5) were introduced, it was thought possible that the whole ulcer problem would be over and that a few weeks' treatment would cure the ulcer for ever. This optimism proved ill-founded, however, when it was discovered that the rate of relapse, recurrence of the ulcer in other words, after treatment with an H_2 antagonist is just as high as if the ulcer has healed of its own accord. So, about 90 per cent of patients suffer from a further attack of ulcer pain within a year of having a course of treatment. This sounds pretty depressing, of course, but it is still the case that the patient has been rapidly relieved of the painful and frightening symptoms on taking the medication.

Doctors have developed various strategies to deal with the problem of relapse and this is something that your doctor will wish to discuss with you. There are sometimes a number of options open to you, and your personal views may be very important in determining the best treatment for you.

Continuous therapy

It is now known that if you take a tablet every single night, this can often keep the ulcer at bay. This is sometimes called continuous therapy. With this sort of treatment about 10 per cent of people will still experience ulcer symptoms during a year's course of drugs – the other 90 per cent, of course, are free of pain and other symptoms.

However, the picture isn't quite as simple as that. Twenty per cent of patients taking continuous medication when examined with an endoscope are found to have ulcers. Whereas half of this group of 20 have ulcer pain, the other half do not: they have what is known as asymptomatic ulcers – ulcers without symptoms. It is eighty, therefore, not ninety, who are actually free of ulcers in any group of 100.

One of the things that scientists have yet to discover is whether or not such asymptomatic ulcers are just as likely to bleed and to perforate as untreated ulcers – in other words how likely they are to develop complications. Even if an ulcer occurs in someone who is taking continuous treatment, it usually responds very rapidly if the dose of tablets is increased from just one at night to two (one at night plus one in the morning).

Surprisingly, there are considerable advantages all round from such a medical approach. Even though tablets are expensive, the amount of time lost off work because of recurrent ulceration is probably a greater economic loss to the country than having people taking continuous treatment. However, many patients are naturally reluctant to take any sort of tablet on a continuous basis – and as soon as they feel well there is a great tendency to forget to take the treatment. This is unfortunate because the ulcer may not have completely healed, despite the absence of pain and other symptoms, and relapse is then rather likely.

Problems with continuous therapy

In many ways the H_2 antagonists are almost perfect drugs in the sense that the side-effects are extremely few and there are no known long-term unpleasant side-effects from taking these drugs continuously. One of the things against taking drugs long-term like this is that it can be some years before what are called idiosyncratic side-effects appear. Idiosyncratic in this context means that the doctors researching and testing the drugs could not possibly have expected those particular side-effects to have developed, given the type of drugs that they were.

Perhaps the best-known example of this is a drug called

Practolol, which was very similar to a safe drug that had been in use for many, many years. Despite this similarity, Practolol after many years' use, was found, quite rarely, to cause a severe fibrosis of the gut, a very dangerous condition. This sort of idiosyncratic side-effect is now very unlikely with the H_2 antagonists which have been prescribed for many years to many millions of patients. However, because of this possibility, many doctors, rather than give continuous treatment, would rather give intermittent therapy. Once an ulcer has been diagnosed for the first time, the patient will almost certainly realize within a few days when it has recurred because of a recurrence of very similar pain and very similar symptoms.

How can you tell if it comes back?

It is worth remembering that when you have had the pain once, if your ulcer comes back you will quickly recognize it, as the pain on recurrence is nearly always very similar. This means that you can go to your doctor and get a further supply of tablets without too much bother. Providing that the original ulcer was a duodenal ulcer, this is pretty safe. If the original ulcer was a gastric ulcer, however, there is a tiny chance that this could be a cancerous gastric ulcer, as described at the end of Chapter 5. Because of this faint possibility, the likelihood of which increases if you are over 50, you should have an endoscopy before taking any further treatment.

What's best?

In general terms, if you are going to have only one or two attacks of pain a year, taking tablets for just six weeks when the pain occurs seems more reasonable than taking tablets all the time. However, some people appear to develop pain almost immediately on stopping the tablets after their six weeks' course. If this happens on several occasions after attempting to stop, it is usually worthwhile having continuous treatment. Incidentally, such patients are *much* more likely to be smokers than non-smokers.

Who relapses and who doesn't?

Unfortunately for doctors, relapsing very rapidly on one occasion after a course of medicine does not necessarily mean that you will do so next time. It is not possible therefore to predict who will relapse and who won't. Doctors cannot divide their patients into rapid relapsers who require continuous therapy and occasional relapsers who clearly do not. It's more a case of trial and error. So, because it is difficult to know how long continuous therapy should be maintained, most doctors would give it for one or two years without attempting to stop. They would then have a go at stopping the tablets to see whether or not the patient finds that the pain rapidly returns. If the pain does return, the doctor would advise the patient to continue with the medication for a further year.

Complications

Certain complications of an ulcer would make it more likely that you should have continuous therapy. Perforation and pyloric stenosis (described in Chapter 2) both mean that you will have to have an operation. The third complication, bleeding, can be treated with a blood transfusion, however, and the bleeding will stop spontaneously. Clearly, with these particular people, it is very important for the doctor to make sure that the ulcer is healed and, if at all possible, stays healed. It is therefore likely that these patients will have continuous treatment for a period of at least one or two years. Specialist advice from a hospital consultant is often needed in order to form an assessment of how long this period should be – you should not accept long-term medication from your GP until you have been seen by a hospital specialist and thoroughly investigated.

The mucosal strengthening agent, De Nol, described in Chapter 5, is thought to help prevent relapse. After a year of treatment some 45–50 per cent of people treated with De Nol relapse, compared with more than 90 per cent if treated with cimetidine. De Nol also seems to work just as well in smokers as in non-smokers, and, indeed, this may be almost entirely responsible for the improved rate of relapse. In other words, the smokers are prevented from relapsing with De Nol, whereas the relapse rate between cimetidine and De Nol in non-smokers is pretty similar.

Clearly, some of us don't want to put up with continuous medicine even though it keeps us well and free of ulcers. A small proportion of ulcer patients, less than 5 per cent, have to have surgery because of complications. A further small percentage, perhaps 10 per cent, many of whom are smokers, continue to have ulcer pain despite various courses of treatment. These patients will undergo surgery.

The various sorts of operation for ulcer patients were described in Chapter 5, but it is worth recapping here while we are talking about the possibility of your ulcer recurring. In a partial gastrectomy of the stomach, the part of the stomach that secretes gastrin is removed. This gastrin tends to stimulate gastric acid and the amount of gastric acid produced after a partial gastrectomy therefore goes down. It goes down partly because of the removal of gastrin and also because part of the acid-secreting portion of the stomach is removed.

This operation has a very low recurrence rate, certainly less than 1 per cent. However, it probably has the highest incidence of side-effects, of the order of some 30 per cent. These vary from a relatively minor problem like being able to eat only a small meal and some weight loss due to anaemia which can be corrected by iron, folic acid or B_{12} injections, to much more serious problems like an increased risk of cancer twenty years later and quite disabling diarrhoea.

The diarrhoea tends to occur for two reasons. First, there is too much fat in the faeces and, secondly, for reasons that are not clearly understood, the partial gastrectomy allows bacteria to grow in the small intestine (there usually aren't any there) and these bacteria ferment the various food products and lead to diarrhoea.

Another rather rare, but nevertheless serious, side-effect occurring after partial gastrectomy is that the bones may become demineralized – in other words, they lose their calcium, and this is because the absorption of calcium is reduced in anyone who has had a partial gastrectomy.

Another operation, vagotomy with drainage procedure (known as pyloroplasty) also produces diarrhoea. This is for two reasons: partly because the gut no longer contracts properly and partly because, again, bacteria can grow in the small intestine where there normally are none and ferment the food and so allow diarrhoea to occur. The recurrence rate with a vagotomy and drainage procedure is much higher than with a partial gastrectomy – it's something like one in ten.

The most sophisticated operation is 'highly selective' vagotomy, in which just the bits of the nerve from the vagus, which is the main nerve feeding the stomach, are cut. This has the highest recurrence rate of all, unfortunately. The rate is greater than one in ten and may be as high as 15 per cent, but, on the other hand, it is the operation that has the lowest incidence of serious side-effects. For those 85 per cent who suffer no recurrence, it is therefore a useful operation.

Playing your part

Whatever the statistics concerning the likely outcome for any particular treatment or surgical procedure, it is true to say that you can improve your own chances by following any drug regime rigorously – don't stop taking the tablets as soon as the pain goes, for the ulcer may not have completely healed and is therefore likely to recur. You can also improve your chances of a rapid return to good health if you do what you can to alter the likelihood of developing an ulcer. If you smoke, for example, you are strongly advised to make every effort to give it up. This, and the other aspects of your lifestyle which may predispose you to developing an ulcer, are discussed in the next chapter.

Hope for the future

The ideal drug would be completely safe, taken for a short course and heal your ulcer for ever. This may be an unrealizable goal, but it is possible that a more complete understanding of the causes of duodenal and gastric ulcers may allow this to happen one day.

A troublesome bug

The organism known as *campylobacter pyloridis*, described in Chapter 5 as part of the case for De Nol, is present in a large number of people with ulcers. It is still not known whether this bug may be there as a coincidental infection or whether it actually causes the ulcer. If it were found to cause ulcers, its eradication could well mean that the ulcer could be healed for good. There may be hope for ulcer patients in the future if current trials provide the hoped for outcome. The bug is known to be sensitive to, in other words adversely affected by, various antibiotics which are in trial stage at the moment to determine whether or not the ulcers heal and whether or not once healed they stay healed. This route to treating ulcers, together with De Nol, are probably the two best possibilities in combating ulcers.

Laser treatments

Another aspect of ulcer treatment which could be improved is the treatment of ulcer bleeding, and for this there are lasers. Lasers are an intense form of light in a thin, parallel beam. A great deal of energy is expended with the impact of a laser

75

upon a surface. If they impact upon a surface of a bleeding artery, lasers can fry the artery with the heat produced by the energy and in this way stop it from further bleeding.

Frying a bleeding ulcer or a bleeding artery with a laser is technically quite difficult for the doctor. He has to be able to see the exact location of the bleeding point through an endoscope; and he has to clear the clot that will have formed over the ulcer in order to expose the artery with the bleeding hole in it.

If the doctor fries the artery too hard, he may fry a hole right through the substance of the stomach and make a hole (a perforation). Happily, with the new forms of laser therapy now available, this is less likely to happen.

Laser therapy is being used now for certain types of bleeding, but its widespread use is at the moment not possible for several reasons. First, the machines are very expensive but their cost should come down as they are more widely used. Second, not all ulcers stop bleeding in response to this type of treatment. Third, it can be difficult to get a straight beam of light located on the ulcer if it is tucked up in a corner of the gut.

Regardless of any problems with lasers, there is little doubt that this type of treatment will before long become a further means of successfully treating ulcers medically – in other words, without surgery – and this would be a valuable advance, particularly for those patients, such as the elderly, who cannot stand up well to an operation.

New drugs

Another hope for the future for ulcer patients is the investigation of various chemicals in the hope of discovering something that mimics the role of one of the body's natural substances, prostaglandin. Prostaglandin is a chemical contained in the blood which, it is thought, may be very important in keeping the mucosal barrier of the stomach strong. If the stomach lining were strengthened in this way, the effect of the acidic gastric juices would be lessened and, conceivably, ulcers wouldn't happen at all. Some synthetic versions of prosta-glandin have been produced, known as methyl-substituted prostaglandins, but as yet they produce results no better than the ulcer drugs currently available and, in addition, are suspected of causing unwanted side-effects.

If these drugs could be refined, and the side-effects elimin-ated, they would have obvious attractions in that they act on the body in a natural way by improving the body's defences. It is not yet clear, however, whether such drugs would also be helpful in preventing ulcers from bleeding and, in addition, preventing the development of ulcers that have been caused by non-steroidal anti-inflammatory drugs, such as aspirin and anti-arthritis drugs.

Avoiding the issue

Whatever hope for the future new drugs extend to the ulcer sufferer, it is certainly the case that preventive medicine is an important part of maintaining good health. The things you can do to keep your body in as good a shape as possible, and therefore more likely to resist the onset of disease, include following a well-balanced nutritious diet, taking meals regu-larly, getting sufficient sleep so that you feel on top of things, taking regular exercise, giving up smoking and cutting down on alcohol and cola drinks. Those measures of preventive medicine that are of particular significance for the ulcer sufferer are described in the next chapter, while those that are generally beneficial are described in Chapter 8.

7

Helping Yourself

Unlike some diseases, having an ulcer is a condition in which you can yourself play a positive part in helping it to heal and preventing another one developing. Natural health practitioners have believed for a long time – and conventional doctors are increasingly realizing – that many diseases are made worse by an unhealthy body and a troubled mind. There is no doubt that regular exercise, attention to maintaining your ideal weight and to keeping your body healthy generally, will increase your resistance to a whole variety of illnesses. There is no reason to suppose that this is not also true of ulcers.

Glancing back over Chapter 4, which described the sort of people who are likely to get an ulcer, will give you lots of clues about the sorts of things you can do – and should not do – to help yourself and your body. Chapter 4 also dealt with the significance of your sex and your age in getting ulcers – but clearly there's nothing you can do about those. The significance of your job was also mentioned – again you may not be able (and you may not want) to do anything about that. You can bring some influence to bear, however, on most of the other factors.

In the family

As ulcers show a small tendency to run in families, it is worth taking all the preventative measures to heart if not only you, but also some of your close relatives, suffer repeatedly with ulcers.

Home

Where you live is not necessarily a crucial issue. Those ulcer sufferers who live in cities only slightly outnumber those who live in rural areas. However, if you live in a busy city area, and you also feel stressed and anxious, it could be worth considering a move to a quieter area.

What you eat

Before your ulcer has been successfully treated (most people respond within two to three weeks of starting the treatment in the case of drugs), you may have noticed an improvement in your symptoms when you eat. About half of all people with ulcers find this. It is sensible, therefore, to eat small amounts frequently through the day so as to keep your stomach more or less continuously buffered from the effects of the acidic digestive juices.

What you eat does not seem to matter very much. We now know that you don't have to stick to white fish (steamed *or* boiled) and that you can eat more or less what you like. With your general health in mind, however, it is best to go for foods that are not too fattening – not too much red meat, cream or butter – and it would be wise to avoid very spicy and highly pickled and peppered dishes.

Fatty, oily foods take longer to digest and therefore stay in the stomach for longer. This means that you may notice that your symptoms are alleviated for longer after fried foods, for example. This does not mean, however, that they are actually good for you – rather the opposite in terms of your general health. Fatty foods are bad for the heart, they clog up your arteries and they also spoil the appearance of your skin.

Many medical conditions are helped greatly by careful attention to diet but this does not appear to be the case with ulcers, the treatments for which are so effective that you can continue to eat more or less normally if you wish. Some people find, however, that virtually all foods upset them when they have an ulcer and they end up drinking tea without sugar and taking dry bread as their only food. This crazy extreme is, of course, far more hazardous to health than continuing to eat two or three curries a day if that happens to be your habit – and curry at least contains meat and vegetables.

Consultant physician Dr Brian Gazzard relates that 'Many of my Indian patients look thoroughly miserable when I see them because they have been off their normal diet for some weeks, often at the insistence of their wife who has read a medical book which is twenty years out of date. The thing that makes them most cheerful is when I tell them that they can go back to eating curries if they like and that this is not harmful. Indeed, most people who come to see me with weird and wonderful diets are much improved by being told to go back and eat what they like. The body often knows what is best and therefore tends to make you wish to eat things that are in fact good for you.'

Stress

Although we know that ulcers can in laboratory conditions be produced in response to stress, and we also know that stress makes the stomach produce more acid, it does not appear to be the case that stress causes the normal chronic peptic ulcer. However, because stress does increase the amount of gastric acid that we secrete, any ulcer will therefore be more painful, and stress could cause any ulceration to increase in severity.

It used to be thought that ulcers were very strongly related to the stress in your life and that they were commoner in the professional classes, the people who were considered to be under more stress than others. It is realized now that it is naive to believe that stress is confined to professional people; it may well be that the stresses caused by shortage of money and unemployment are much worse than the stresses of large business lunches.

Stress itself does not appear to be a very important factor in people developing an ulcer. Many people who are stressed do have ulcers but, equally, many people who are totally phlegmatic and allow everything to flow over them also have ulceration.

Group support

As we saw in Chapter 4, soldiers in both World Wars developed ulcers less when they were placed in stressful situations (such as being a prisoner of war or fighting at the front) than when they were no longer benefiting from the support of their comrades when they returned home. Stress, in other words, played a less important part in the context of ulcers than group exclusion.

This isolation from comrades, peers, friends and so on can be related to the lives of many people. Being a bored housewife with grown up children, or a lone craftsman, for example, could breed feelings of isolation and group exclusion. Much the same sort of thing can happen if you are plucked from a familiar environment and relocated elsewhere, perhaps not as a consequence of your own decision: for example, the wives of diplomats, politicians and bankers can be transferred to Hong Kong or Brussels, for instance, to a totally alien environment with none of their usual support systems. Although it would seem on the face of it that these women have nothing to worry about, they may be far from happy and turn to alcohol and fruitless pursuits. These are people who are temporarily bereft and with not enough to do that interests them who may be stressed in ways that have nothing to do with pressure of time, commitments or lack of money.

The answer in such a situation is to go out and look for what interests you in your environment, and if it is not there to try to create it, obtain it or alternatively turn yourself to entirely new interests. The important thing is to build a network of friends, interests and helpers.

If, on the other hand, you find practically everything about your environment loathsome and you envisage a happier, healthier life elsewhere, it may be that your only course is to move. Whether this would prevent a recurrence of an ulcer is really very debatable, but, as was said at the beginning of this chapter, even conventional doctors are more and more realizing that many diseases are made worse by an unhealthy body and a troubled mind.

81

Your own stress levels

Many doctors believe that the amount of stress in one's life can be reduced by setting aside part of every day for your personal enjoyment, either by various exercises such as simple meditation, sitting in a dark room listening to music, or listening to relaxation tapes. All these things help you to regain some control over your body mechanisms in that you can assess the manifestations of stress by your pulse rate, sweating and general feelings of anxiety. Autogenics, biofeedback and yoga are all useful in this context and these are discussed in Chapter 8.

Drink

Some people find that their ulcer pain is exacerbated by drinking alcohol but most notice practically no effect if the amount of alcohol is small. It is now considered almost certainly not to be harmful to ulcer patients, provided that it is taken in moderation. Obviously, it would not be sensible to drink on an empty stomach nor during an attack of ulcer pain. Now would it be wise to drink a lot.

We have pretty clear guidelines these days for what constitutes 'a lot'. We also know that it is bad for your general health, both physical and mental, to drink too much on a regular basis. 'A lot' – in fact too much – is, for men, 5 to 7 pints a day or 10 glasses of wine (or a litre bottle) a day. For women, 'a lot' is less, partly because of their smaller body and partly because a woman's body appears to make more use of alcohol; what is termed 'take-up' appears to be more efficient and therefore more intoxicating and potentially more dangerous than the same quantity would be for a man. For women, then, a lot is 3½ to 5 pints of beer a day or 7 glasses of wine.

The amount that is regarded by doctors as 'moderate' or 'safe' is 4 pints of beer or 8 glasses of wine *a week* for men; for women it is considered safe to drink 3 pints of beer or 6 glasses of wine each week.

Heavy drinking greatly increases your chances of lasting damage to your body, both physical and mental, including liver disease, ulcers, heart and circulatory disorders and brain damage. Early warning symptoms and signs include impaired memory (a sign of brain damage and irreversible) and the dry heaves. This is the nausea and vomiting that an alcoholic experiences in the morning and is a sure sign of drinking too much. It is related to the inflammation of the stomach caused by the alcohol; ulcers cause another form of stomach inflammation. If you are drinking this much, you ought to cut down whether you have ulcers or not. If you do have ulcers, you *must* cut down.

Caffeine, chiefly in the form of coffee and colas, is thought to cause or exacerbate ulcers. If you have an ulcer, therefore, you would be wise to exclude these drinks from your diet. If you are lucky enough not to have an ulcer, it is worth noting that just two cups of coffee a day doubles your risk of developing an ulcer. If ulcers run in the family and you have blood group O and you smoke, it is recommended that you give up both coffee and smoking.

Smoking

Unlike drinking alcohol, any amount of smoking is dangerously harmful to your health. For the ulcer sufferer it is especially dangerous in that smokers are twice as likely as non-smokers to develop ulcers, they respond less well to treatment and they are more likely to develop complications, such as pyloric stenosis, perforation or haemorrhage (all described in Chapter 2), with their ulcers.

The justifications for giving up smoking are many and powerful: apart from ulcers, other smoking-related diseases include lung cancer (from which 40,000 people die in the UK every year); heart disease, chronic bronchitis, emphysema, cancer of the mouth and throat; cancer of the bowel, angina. The smoking habit kills four times as many people as the total who die by drink, drugs, murder, suicide, road accidents, rail accidents, air accidents, poisoning, drowning, fires, falls, snake bites, lightning and every other cause of accidental death all put together.

If you are a smoker and an ulcer sufferer, the most important thing you can do to help yourself and your body to better health is to kick the habit. Before the Health Education Council was reconstituted and brought under the aegis of the government, it identified four stages in giving up smoking:

1 Thinking about your reasons for stopping.
2 Preparing to stop.
3 Stopping.
4 Staying stopped.

You already know the reasons for stopping, so move on to stage 2. First of all, decide on the day. If your spouse smokes, try to get him or her to agree to stop with you on that particular day. Now go around the house and remove all the paraphernalia – such as ashtrays, cigarettes, lighters, matches, and lighter refills.

The next step is to decide what you are going to do with all the extra time and money you will have on your hands. Taking time first, it is worth organizing things to do, especially in the first few weeks, that will both *prevent* you smoking and also take your mind off it. These include going to the theatre, ballet or opera; swimming and other sports; and seeing friends who are rabid non-smokers. As for money, you could spend it all on theatre tickets or go shopping to reward yourself for giving up, or, perhaps more wisely, calculate how much you have been spending on cigarettes each month (it could well be £100 a month) and divert all this into a separate account. Decide what you will do with that extra £1000 after a year or so. And if there's two of you, the sum could be closer to £2500 by the end of the 12 months.

So far, it has all been comparatively easy planning. The next step in stage 2 is practice. If you are smoking more than say 15 a day, you need to cut down, just like any other drug, before you cut yourself off. One way of cutting down is to cut down on the areas in which you can smoke. Declare the bedroom the first No Smoking zone, for instance. Then add the bathroom, followed by the kitchen. Work your way through the rooms that you habitually use, including your office or wherever you work. Another way of cutting down is by doing things that don't allow you to smoke at the same time, such as theatre trips or swimming as described earlier.

A third method, and this is said to be particularly effective, is to put back the time of day that you start smoking so that it is later and later each day. The reason that this is said to be effective is that experts have discovered that the earlier in the day you smoke, the greater the frequency of smoking will be in the day. So it's not just that you have smoked fewer cigarettes because you allocated fewer hours in the day to smoking, but that the number of cigarettes you light up each hour will decrease the later you start.

You are now nearing the day on which you are going to stop. You are down to some 5 or 10, all of which you smoke in the living room or garden. You may have been finding it difficult to concentrate (a sign of withdrawal from nicotine) and you may have had stomach cramps and an unpleasant taste in the mouth. You will find that these things will clear up not too long after you have given up, however.

The day itself arrives and you are about to release yourself from an addiction that is a danger to you and offensive to many others. Keep yourself busy. Start off with a good breakfast and lots of orange juice to get rid of the nasty taste in your mouth. If you are going to work, make sure that there's lots to do. If you've settled on a weekend, do what you enjoy most, whether it's gardening, going to the sea, shopping, visiting an art gallery, playing tennis or cards. If you find after dinner that your resolve is being threatened, go to bed early. The next day will be better and you will already have one day's experience of your new status as a non-smoker.

There's no doubt that the first few weeks of giving up, particularly for a heavy smoker, are not easy. Your body is demanding the drug to which it is addicted and you have to hold out. Some people don't get too many withdrawal symptoms. If you do, keep reminding yourself that this is simply a short phase while your body adjusts and releases the deposits that have been built up. If you find yourself feeling depressed, irritable, impatient or anxious, bear in mind that these are all symptoms of withdrawal and that they will disappear within a short time. Fight these on a day-to-day basis with the satisfaction of knowing that the addiction is weakening its grip upon you as time goes by.

Other drugs

If you are taking other drugs which may reduce the effectiveness of the drugs you have been given for ulcers, or indeed drugs that are believed to cause ulceration, discuss the subject fully with your doctor (this is discussed more fully in Chapter 5). It should be stressed here that if you feel your anti-arthritis drugs, for example, are not actually doing much to relieve the discomfort, you should consider substituting them with something such as paracetamol, which is believed not to damage the stomach lining.

Aspirin is thought to damage the lining of the gut when taken continuously in large doses. The same applies, of course, to those over-the-counter painkillers that contain aspirin. If you find that you need to take painkillers on a regular basis, whether it is for a headache or whatever, you are advised to use paracetamol particularly if you are disposed to getting ulcers.

Monitoring your health

Health pundits and writers often encourage people to make lists or charts of their condition and their symptoms together with the time of day that the symptoms manifest themselves most strongly. Most doctors, however, secretly heave a sigh of horror when a chart or detailed list of symptoms is produced in the consulting room. This is because such lists in many ways make the diagnosis more difficult for the doctor. The doctor is interested in the overall story that a patient produces, in which the details are forgotten. It is usually the most important symptoms that stick in the patient's mind. The disadvantage of writing everything down is that it does not indicate to the doctor the importance or severity of each individual symptom.

In addition, everyone has all sorts of aches and pains in the chest and in the stomach now and again. Most of us, when we have an ulcer, will know that there is something quite different about the intensity, duration, location and the quality of the pain.

Generally speaking, it is rather obsessional people who make detailed charts of everything and often get themselves into a panic about comparatively minor symptoms. Your doctor will probably appreciate that many people are anxious when they consult him or her and that they may be nervous and forgetful. You should be reassured, however, that the doctor will question you in order to establish the significant facts and almost certainly the things that you have forgotten to tell him or her are not of any real significance. Diagnoses are nearly always made on the basis of a combination of symptom patterns and so, although the doctor's questioning may strike you as rather random, in reality he or she is probing to see whether other symptoms will fit in with this diagnosis. Various odd symptoms that the patient may have experienced, such as a tingling in the nose, or itchy feet, associated with stomach pain, are not likely to be relevant. The fact that these minor symptoms are forgotten in the consulting room because they have not been committed to a list doesn't really matter very much.

Your health plan

This chapter has concentrated on the most important aspects of self-help for the person who has an ulcer. There are other aspects of good health, however, which all of us, including the ulcer sufferer, may benefit from applying. These are the things that can help all of us increase our body's resistance to disease including ulcer disease. These measures of preventive medicine are described in Chapter 8.

8

Preventing Ulcers

If you want to prevent an ulcer developing, says consultant physician Dr Brian Gazzard, 'the rather unrealistic thing you can do is to spend the rest of your life in a large group of people with whom you have lots in common, chewing chapattis, in rural northern India, never smoking, drinking moderate amounts of alcohol but not taking any aspirin for the hangover that results. Not many of us can do this, of course, although the idea of life on an ashram may be quite attractive.'

Dr Gazzard has picked on certain aspects of our health and lifestyle and identified those things that are of particular relevance to the classic ulcer sufferer, described in Chapter 4. That chapter offered a number of clues to how you can prevent an ulcer recurring and Chapter 7 concentrated on how you can put into practice ways of reducing the likelihood of the problem returning. Chief among these is giving up smoking, trying to find substitutes for drugs such as aspirin and anti-arthritis pills and cutting down on alcohol and cola drinks.

There is quite a lot more that you can do to improve your general health, however, and this applies not only to those of us who would like to prevent any further ulcers developing but also to those of us who may not have had an ulcer but wish to improve the healthy functioning of the body and the mind in order to increase the body's resistance to disease. Ways in which you can make yourself healthier include sensible diet, maintaining your ideal weight, sleep, exercise and relaxation.

What you eat

Most things will not do your ulcer much harm. What might make it worse is suddenly to alter your diet dramatically. All you need to remember is to avoid very fatty and fried foods, and spicy peppery or pickled foods. For good general health it is best to eat a varied diet, selecting foods from the four main groups each day.

Group 1 includes protein in the form of meat, fish and eggs. Avoid fatty things like goose, duck, herring and mackerel. Red meats, such as beef and lamb, are best eaten only once or twice a week. Concentrate instead on chicken, pork and lots of fish – plaice, cod, halibut and trout, for example. All these things are best grilled, boiled, casseroled or poached – do avoid frying.

Group 2 comprises the dairy products of cheese, butter, cream and milk. All these things contain a lot of fat but, on the other hand. they are also good for you. Milk is particularly useful for ulcer sufferers as it buffers the acid in the stomach; however, its goodness is in the watery part, not the creamy part. This means that you do not need full cream milk and, in fact, skimmed milk would be a lot healthier both for the ulcer sufferer and the rest of us. With good health in mind, cream ought to be avoided altogether and cheese and butter taken very sparingly. You can halve your consumption of butter at breakfast, for example, by eating one large slice of wholemeal bread, buttered, instead of two. Using margarine and other vegetable fats, particularly in cooking, is much healthier than using butter. Lastly, unsalted butter is better for you than salted butter.

Group 3 foods include all vegetables and fruits, which are all good for you to a greater or lesser degree. Green vegetables, particularly spinach, are a good source of vitamins. Oranges come top of the fruit league, but ulcer sufferers may find that any acidic fruits, such as grapefruit and lemon, may upset them. Apples are also very good, but you may find that you want to avoid Granny Smiths and choose something a bit less acidic, such as Coxes or Golden Delicious. It is recommended that you eat fruit and vegetables in some form twice a day, every day.

The last group of foods, Group 4, includes cereals, pulses and grains, which supply most of the fibre we eat. Fibre in the diet is important for all of us and is believed to be particularly important for ulcer sufferers although this has not yet been definitively proved. You can get it in the form of wholewheat cereals, bran-based cereals, muesli, beans and baked beans, wholewheat and granary bread, bran biscuits, wholemeal pitta bread, wholewheat spaghetti and other types of pasta, including macaroni, shells and lasagne. So, as you can see, there's no shortage of foods to fit the fibre bill – you don't have to take the unpalatable step of sprinkling a tablespoon or two of bran over your cereal unless you happen to like it.

As for drinks, your best bets are milk, fruit juices, milky tea, peppermint tea or China teas such as Earl Grey.

The foods you ought to avoid, if you don't want to feel sluggish and your arteries to be clogged, are sweets, chocolate, most biscuits, cakes, buns, lashings of Double Devon clotted cream, oils as in salad dressings, sardines and tuna in oil, peanut butter, alcoholic drinks, and traditional English breakfasts with fried bread oozing fat. You don't need any one of these things for health – they are extras in the diet which you can, of course, eat from time to time but they should not feature regularly in your weekly diet.

Fortunately, ulcer sufferers no longer have to stick to boring and restrictive diets, and so you have complete freedom of choice provided you choose foods chiefly from the four main food groups.

Best bets for breakfast are muesli or a bran-based cereal with fruit, apple juice, milky tea and a slice or two of wholemeal or granary bread with margarine and marmalade. Lunch could be a leek quiche on a wholemeal pastry base with baked potato and a large salad (no butter on the potato and the smallest amount of salad dressing!). If you have to have sandwiches, try and get wholemeal or granary bread and avoid salami, tuna, cream cheese; choose instead chicken, salmon, cottage cheese or hardboiled egg without mayonnaise.

Dinner is easier in that you will probably have more time to think about the four food groups and make your choice: remember the fibre content chiefly, and substitute fruit or yogurt (or both) for puddings. Skip after-dinner coffee as this really does adversely affect ulcer sufferers and it doesn't do the rest of us much good, either. Coffee is quite a powerful stimulant and it is also addictive, as you will discover if you stop, having been used to drinking four or five mugs of coffee a day. Caffeine withdrawal is characterized by headaches, drowsiness and poor concentration, but this temporary phase soon passes if you stick it out.

The advantages of a healthy diet as described over the last page or two are many, the most noticeable of which is that you will soon find you have lots more energy and feel generally more alert and fit.

If you need to lose weight, the best method, and the method with which all doctors agree, is to follow a well-balanced diet, taking food each day from the four main groups in smaller quantities than you are used to. If you usually eat two baked potatoes at dinner, cut down to one. If you normally eat two rounds of sandwiches and a chocolate bar at lunchtime, eat just one round and an apple. Never cut breakfast – it's much better to halve the amount that you eat in the evening, when you will need less energy, than it is to skimp at the start of the day. Above all, do not go for faddy commercial diets, whether they are ones that substitute powders and milk drinks for foods or ones that say you've got to eat lamb and pears, or steak and grapefruit, for days or weeks on end. These are potentially dangerous diets – and particularly so if you are already not in full health. These are diets promoted by people whose business it is to make money – they are not interested in your health.

Calorie-counting diets are not particularly helpful for health, either, and this is because they do not take account of the fact that many foods that are extremely nutritious, such as meat, fish and cheese, are also high in calories: a calorie is a unit of measurement of energy, not of fat. Things such as sugar, which you will notice does not qualify for inclusion in any of the four food groups, are high in calories and can be excluded completely from the diet. The fruit that you eat will provide you with more than enough sugar for energy.

Lastly, a look at so-called junk food. Let's look at hamburgers and chips: you've got minced beef shaped into a burger and fried, together with a white bread bun and fried potatoes. The minced beef will not be pure – various other unusable parts of the animal will be minced with the beef, it is fried in oil, the bun is not wholemeal and the potatoes have been fried in oil, the most nutritious part having been removed (the goodness lies just beneath the skin, which is why baked potatoes are good for you). If you were to make your own grilled burgers at home, put them in a wholemeal bun and serve with a baked potato and a large salad, you would have a meal that is twice as good for you. Alternatively, a chicken salad sandwich on wholemeal bread, followed by an apple, would be a better choice for a quick meal than a burger and chips.

One of the problems with junk or convenience foods is not necessarily that they contain harmful additives as the fact that they rarely contain enough of what's good for you. Vitamin content will have been severely reduced in the cooking and storage methods, and the fibre content is likely to be low. As for the concept of convenience, nothing could be more convenient than a cheese and tomato wholemeal sandwich and an apple – and it's cheap as well. If you are at home, another quick and convenient meal containing all the nourishment you need is baked beans on wholemeal toast with a poached egg on top.

Sleep

Nothing revitalizes the mind and the body so well as the right amount of sleep taken on a regular basis. The occasional late night doesn't do any harm but what you need to avoid is habitually staying up too late, getting too tired and waking up late in the morning and having to rush. You probably know how many hour's sleep you feel best with – some people function well with as little as five or six hours, while others habitually need at least nine – and this is what you should be aiming to get. So fight the compulsion to start some work or a house job at 11 at night and don't be tempted to stay up and watch second-rate movies on television. You will find if you go to bed a little bit earlier, you will be able to achieve much more the following day.

If your body is over-tired and worn out, it will find it much harder to fight illness and disease, including ulcers.

Exercise

The rewards of regular exercise are many. You will feel more alert, you will be able to achieve more, you will also feel more relaxed afterwards and, like an engine, your body will benefit from a proper workout, changing its status to that of a finely tuned engine from the sluggish old motor of yesterday.

What sort of exercise you take depends on what you like. Exercising every day is an ideal, but if time is short three 20-minute periods of exercise a week should be enough to keep you fit. Swimming is by far the best all-round exercise, but if that's not convenient, choose between running, brisk walking, or tennis. Golf is really too leisurely to count, although the fresh air will do you good, and squash is too demanding while you have a painful ulcer. If you decide that walking is as much exercise as you feel like taking, remember that you should set yourself a fairly brisk pace. Ambling doesn't count!

You can increase the amount of exercise you get, and the amount of fresh air, by altering your everyday habits a little. For example, walk up stairs rather than take a lift or escalator. Walk on to the next bus stop and get off one earlier than the one you need. If you live no more than 20 minutes' walk, say, from the shops, walk instead of driving. If you live or work in a busy city, you may be surprised to find that you can get from A to B more quickly by walking than by waiting for a bus or descending hundreds of steps into the Tube.

Relaxation

Exercise will make you feel more relaxed but it is also important to set aside some time each day for quiet, gentle relaxation and contemplation. You may find that the best way for you is to sit in a darkened room, listening to music, or you may find that one of the less strenuous aspects of gardening, for example, is more effective. Reading is another option and some of what are known as the alternative therapies are others.

It is extremely unlikely that any of the alternative therapies – which include acupuncture, Alexander Technique, healing, herbalism, homoeopathy, hypnotherapy, massage, meditation, osteopathy, reflexology and yoga – could prevent an ulcer developing. It is also doubtful whether any of these therapies could cause an ulcer to heal, although it should be noted that an ulcer will often heal of its own accord given time. That makes it rather difficult to judge the efficacy of such treatments when applied to ulcer patients.

Although the alternative health systems may not be able to heal an ulcer and they are even more unlikely to help the patient who has ulcer complications (which should be regarded as a medical emergency), many people have benefited in a general sense, both psychologically and physically, when treated by one or other of these methods. Alternative health practitioners believe that the body has the power to fight disease and that this power can be encouraged by such systems. They also believe that the drugs prescribed by conventional doctors are all more or less harmful to some degree and serve to deal only with the symptoms of disease rather than the cause. All this is highly debatable, however.

The sensible compromise for the ulcer sufferer seems to be to take medical drugs as prescribed for the full course and at the same time to follow such alternative systems as seem attractive. Some alternative health specialists are also qualified doctors who will have the letters MD or MB after their name, and these may be your best bet. If someone calls himself or herself a doctor, but the letters after their name are PhD, this means that they hold a doctorate, not that they are qualified in medicine as doctors. It is also worth checking that the practitioner you choose is a member of his/her professional association.

Acupuncture

This may give the ulcer patient some remission of pain but it is thought unlikely to make the ulcer heal itself.

Alexander Technique

This is a system of postural and relaxation exercises, which should help you to relax and may reduce pain but will not heal the ulcer.

Healing

Healers have had spectacular results from time to time and, if you are lucky, you may find that your ulcer goes away, never to return. This obviously cannot be considered a reliable method of treatment, however.

Herbalism

Many drugs in use by conventional doctors are synthetic derivatives of versions of the natural substances that the herbalist uses. Herbalism includes in its repertoire a number of infusions and decoctions that can be used to relieve inflammation and pain and could therefore be helpful to the ulcer patient. Stronger drugs may be needed for a complete cure, however.

Homoeopathy

Quite a few homoeopaths are qualified doctors, so you should be able to find one who understands the nature of ulcer disease. The homoeopath should, at least, be able to relieve pain, inflammation and flatulence. He or she will also be able to prescribe sleeping draughts if ulcer pain is causing you to wake during the night.

Hypnotherapy

Hypnosis can help the ulcer patient only in learning to relax, and this alone, although helpful, is unlikely to make the ulcer heal.

Massage

This can be recommended as a luxurious and enjoyable treatment with short-term benefits of relaxation, provided that the stomach and abdominal area is avoided.

Meditation

Again, this is useful as a way of learning to relax.

Osteopathy

This is concerned with the skeleton of the body, the bones and muscles, and has little to offer the ulcer patient. Its advocates claim that such therapy can improve the nerve supplies to the stomach and thus help the healing of ulcers.

Reflexology

Pain relief is the chief attraction for the ulcer sufferer.

Yoga

Once again, this a therapy that is useful in teaching you to relax, and as such has a positive and beneficial effect, particularly if you set aside some time regularly each day. In common with the other alternative systems, however, it is not thought to be able to cure ulcers, nor to prevent them developing.

Alternative preventive measures

Because simple ulcers heal of their own accord in time, it is very difficult to determine the effect of any particular natural health option. It is also impossible to say whether or not these options could prevent an ulcer developing. Some doctors believe that these symptoms do help keep people in good health, partly because they nearly all teach you to relax and partly because their practitioners are almost always firm advocates of a healthy way of life. This is usually regarded as part of the treatment and practitioners will therefore promote a healthy diet, as described earlier in this chapter (with the exception that some will recommend excluding meat and fish); adequate sleep; regular exercise; and urge you to give up smoking, drinking, caffeine, and white sugar. All this is good and should be regarded as part of your health plan, whether you are an ulcer patient or not.

Keeping an eye on things

Taking good care of yourself can do much to prevent the return of an ulcer, but it is worth keeping an eye on things. Always go for the check-ups suggested by your GP or your consultant, and always take any tablets for the entire course, even if the pain stops quite quickly. Pain is only one symptom; the fact that it stops does not necessarily mean that the ulcer is completely healed. Lastly, if you experience any of the familiar symptoms of pain, nausea and vomiting, loss of appetite or bleeding (either in the vomit or in the faeces), do consult your doctor without delay. Any condition that is treated early on is more likely to be cured more quickly; your body will be given a greater chance of resisting the disease and perhaps you'll prevent your ulcer coming back.

Index

Figures in *italics* refer to diagrams

99